Law and Ethics
for the Eye Care Professional

Law and Ethics
for the Eye Care Professional

Barbara K Pierscionek BSc (Optom) PhD MBA
Postgrad Dip (Law) (LLB equiv) Postgrad Dip
(Legal Practice) LLM

Professor of Optometry and Vision Science,
Department of Biomedical Sciences,
University of Ulster, Coleraine

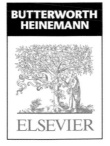

Edinburgh   London   New York   Oxford
Philadelphia   St Louis   Sydney   Toronto   2008

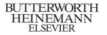

OPTO
.016498185

BUTTERWORTH
HEINEMANN
ELSEVIER

Notice

Knowledge and best practice in this field are constantly changing. As new research and experience broaden our knowledge, changes in practice, treatment and drug therapy may become necessary or appropriate. Readers are advised to check the most current information provided (i) on procedures featured or (ii) by the manufacturer of each product to be administered, to verify the recommended dose or formula, the method and duration of administration, and contraindications. It is the responsibility of the practitioner, relying on their own experience and knowledge of the patient, to make diagnoses, to determine dosages and the best treatment for each individual patient, and to take all appropriate safety precautions. To the fullest extent of the law, neither the publisher nor the author assumes any liability for any injury and/or damage.

The Publisher

OP TO
Mylar

First published 2008
ISBN: 978-0-08-045033-9

British Library Cataloguing in Publication Data
A catalogue record for this book is available from the British Library

Library of Congress Cataloging in Publication Data
A catalog record for this book is available from the Library of Congress

For Elsevier:
Commissioning Editor: Robert Edwards
Development Editor: Rebecca Gleave
Project Manager: Susan Stuart
Designer: Sarah Russell

Printed in China

The Publisher's policy is to use paper manufactured from sustainable forests

Working together to grow
libraries in developing countries

www.elsevier.com | www.bookaid.org | www.sabre.org

ELSEVIER　　BOOK AID
International　　Sabre Foundation

12/05/08
pgm

Contents

RE
959
P52
2008
OPTO

Preface vii

Acknowledgements viii

About the author ix

Chapter 1   Introduction to ethics 1

Chapter 2   Professions 19

Chapter 3   The optometric code of ethics and basic ethical concepts 33

Chapter 4   Beneficence/non-maleficence 49

Chapter 5   Respect for autonomy 65

Chapter 6   Justice 85

Chapter 7   Confidentiality/data protection 103

Chapter 8   Collegiality and employment law 122

Chapter 9   The tort of negligence 142

Chapter 10   Business ethics 161

Chapter 11   Ethical dilemmas 174

Chapter 12   Philosophy and ethical theory 188

Index 204

Preface

This book is intended to introduce basic ethical and legal principles to the eye care practitioner. It was not intended to provide detailed and prescriptive measures for tackling ethical problems, as there is no single right way to do this and every practitioner needs to develop their own ethical approach. The book offers scope for reflection and for broadening perspectives beyond the consulting room.

Examples included have, wherever possible, been taken from life: current affairs, real situations, my own experiences in academia and practice, and the personal experiences that others have related to me.

This is a handbook as much for the undergraduate student who is about to embark on a career in optometry and health care as for the experienced practitioner who wishes to refresh or further his or her knowledge of ethics and the relevant law.

Barbara Krystyna Pierscionek
July 2007

Acknowledgements

A heartfelt thank you to two very special people: my son Tomasz Pierscionek for all that his empathy and insights have taught me and Dr Hans Bruun for his patience, good humour and faith.

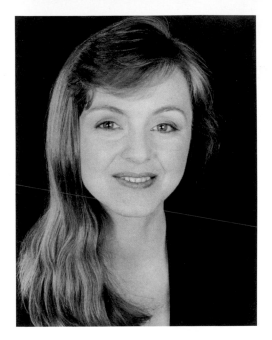

Barbara Krystyna Pierscionek was born in London, England, where she spent her formative years. She has lived in Australia and completed her first two degrees at the University of Melbourne. After graduating with a PhD in biochemistry and optics, she continued studies on the eye and changes with age as an independent researcher funded by the Australian Medical Research Council (NHMRC). Shortly after returning to the United Kingdom she completed an MBA and obtained legal qualifications, including the theoretical degree required to practise as a solicitor in England and Wales as well as a Master's degree in Law (LLM). She currently holds a Chair in the Department of Biomedical Sciences at the University of Ulster where she teaches healthcare ethics and law, and researches in rheology, optics and biochemistry of the eye as well as on emerging ethical and legal issues in medicine and health care.

1

Introduction to ethics

WHAT IS THE MEANING OF ETHICS?

Ethics appears in a vast range of disciplines – from philosophy to politics, from medicine to science. The question 'What does ethics mean?' can elicit a number of answers, each as individual as the respondent. The reason for this is that a simple definition of ethics does not exist – perhaps because the concept has been around for more than two millennia and its meaning and application have been altered and reinterpreted with time and according to culture. Or perhaps because we can never impose a strict definition on an aspect of human behaviour that is rooted in morality.

The ancient Greeks treated ethics as defining good deeds. Aristotle believed that all human actions aim for some good. He used *ethike* to mean moral virtue that comes from good habits. The concept of duty has also been introduced to describe ethics. The great philosopher, Immanuel Kant, believed that our actions and ethical behaviour do not stem from wanting purely to do good, but rather from a sense of duty, and that this duty and how to fulfil it comes from human reason.

As, according to Kant, ethical behaviour comes from reason there should surely be a common moral law and hence a universal set of ethical principles? Many others have found this prospect unattainable and the debates about definitions of ethics are interminable. Yet, the need to find a strict definition of ethics may not be necessary because ethical principles are not a set of fixed rules with rigid definitions. Ethical principles are guidelines that help a person to make decisions and to justify why and how these decisions have led to certain actions. The decisions and actions may vary depending on the situation but the basic principles should remain the same. The practice of ethics requires careful thought, questioning and justification of choices, decisions and actions.

Some decisions are easy. Should you increase a prescription that is more than 2 years old by a small amount such as 0.5D? Although this is only a slight change in prescription, the patient may prefer to have this change. Alternatively, a patient may be happy enough to continue with their old pair of spectacles. If visual acuity through the old prescription is sufficient for daily needs and not under any legal limit, the decision may be not to prescribe a new pair of spectacles. Such situations, which require relatively straightforward decisions, occur frequently in healthcare practice. Less frequent are situations in which the decisions that need to be made are so difficult that the healthcare or medical practitioner has to seek help to decide what to do.

There are situations in which what may appear to be a simple question can, in fact, be one for which no simple or even acceptable answer is available. If anyone were asked whether it is wrong to kill a baby, the answer, for most people, would be vehemently in the affirmative. Yet when that question was put into the context of a difficult situation, such as the one faced by doctors treating the conjoined twins, Mary and Jodie, the answer was not clear (Re A (Children) [2000]). In this case the twins were born joined at the lower pelvis with a fusion of the lower spines. Although each twin had her own vital organs, Mary's brain was poorly developed; her heart was enlarged and malfunctioning, and she had very little functional lung tissue. Jodie's vital organs were working well and Mary was kept alive only because Jodie was supplying her with oxygenated blood. The doctors treating the infants claimed that this situation was not sustainable for either child. Jodie's organs could not continue to keep Jodie and Mary alive for more than a very short period. In order to save Jodie's life, the doctors claimed that they would need to separate the twins, but the operation would surely kill Mary. This was a case unprecedented in medical and legal history. Legal, ethical and moral arguments for and against the operation were presented and each had its merits and its problems. The answer to whether or not an operation that would result in the death of a child should be conducted was anything but simple. The case went to the courts and it was decided that the twins should be separated. The transcripts of the Law Lords, whose responsibility it was to decide the fate of these two infants, showed the difficulty that each had with making the decision that he made (Re A (Children) [2000]).

In eye care practice, there are no such life and death decisions to be made, but it is possible that sight-threatening cases may arise. There may be no guidelines or laws to give directions and the onus is on practitioners to make decisions that they may find difficult. Whatever is decided, practitioners will have to be able to justify those decision, to themselves, to colleagues and, if necessary, to the public.

Often the hardest decisions to make are those that offer two or more outcomes, none of which is entirely satisfactory:

Clinical case study

One of your best friends is a patient at your practice. You have been good friends since school and share many experiences and memories. You can count on and confide in one another. One day your friend comes in for a routine examination and you notice that something is not right with his demeanour and manner. He is clearly distressed but reluctant to discuss it. Eventually, during the course of the examination, he asks you whether you can keep secret something that he desperately needs to tell someone. He has felt for years that he is a homosexual and only recently has he accepted this. The reason he took so much time to come to terms with it was because of his staunchly conservative upbringing. He is sure that his parents would never accept it and he has to keep it a secret. You are a little surprised with the revelation but you make no judgement and promise to keep this secret.

This is, however, not the whole story. Your friend has had a relationship with a partner who has been diagnosed with AIDS and your friend suspects that he too may be affected. He has not yet had this confirmed. You promise to keep this to yourself and to offer him any support he may need, whatever the diagnosis. Your friend leaves at the end of the examination. Two days later you hear from his sister that he died from a heart attack. It is then that you remember your friend had offered to donate organs, including his corneae. His sister confirms that his wish to donate his organs will be honoured.

Would you keep your friend's secret?

THE HISTORY OF ETHICS IN HEALTH CARE

In health care, the ethical principles we use today are founded on the oath of Hippocrates. Hippocrates lived around 460–380 BC and was thought to be a member of a cult of physicians who were faithful to Asclepius (or Aesculepius, the Roman version), the god of medicine and healing. The symbol of the medical profession – a snake wrapped around a physician's staff – is attributed to Asclepius. Snakes may appear to be an unusual symbol for medicine and health care today, but they were vital for the healing rituals in ancient Greece. Non-poisonous snakes were put into rooms where the sick slept on the ground. Some of the myths about Asclepius suggest a deeper understanding of healthcare ethics by the ancients than is often acknowledged. For example, the reason for Asclepius' death, by the hand of the god Zeus, is sometimes cited when technological advances in medicine are thought by some to have transgressed too far. Asclepius was killed by a thunderbolt sent by Zeus, because Asclepius had resurrected a dead man. As Asclepius was half mortal, Zeus did not think it right that a mortal should bring another mortal back from the dead, for this was not in the realm of men.

The same sentiment resonates today when the argument is made that doctors and scientists should not 'play God'. Recent cases of babies born prematurely or with severe deformities are examples of when such arguments have been raised. Technology has given doctors greater powers but is it always right to use these powers?

The case of Charlotte Wyatt

Charlotte Wyatt was born 12 weeks prematurely and she weighed just one pound. She had to be fed through a tube and required oxygen supplied by artificial means. The doctors who were treating Charlotte, and who had to resuscitate her on more than one occasion, did not think it was in her best interests to keep doing so because her quality of life was deemed to be so poor. She had severe brain, lung and kidney damage. In the past such premature children had no chance of survival but scientific and technological advances now allow maintenance of life for so fragile an infant by artificial means.

The ethical debates that arose around the case of baby Charlotte were generally centred around this issue: sustaining life at all and at any cost

Continued

against letting nature take its course (Re Wyatt [2004]). Interestingly, baby Charlotte, originally given months to live, defied all predictions and, when she was 2 years old, the judge held that it should be ultimately up to the doctors to make the decision about whether to not to resuscitate her (Re Wyatt [2006]). The issues of best interests, quality of life and whether or not a premature infant should be given every opportunity to live, even if that requires artificial means, are left to doctors (and judges) to decide. The decisions do not always follow the course that Nature may have taken, if allowed to do so.

The Hippocratic Oath

The original oath written by Hippocrates has several translations. The version of Chadwick & Mann (1950) is shown below:

"I swear by Apollo the healer, by Aesculapius, by Health and all the powers of healing, and call to witness all the gods and goddesses that I may keep this Oath and Promise to the best of my ability and judgement.

I will pay the same respect to my master in the Science as to my parents and share my life with him and pay all my debts to him. I will regard his sons as my brothers and teach them the Science, if they desire to learn it, without fee or contract. I will hand on precepts, lectures and all other learning to my sons, to those of my master and to those pupils duly apprenticed and sworn, and to none other.

I will use my power to help the sick to the best of my ability and judgement; I will abstain from harming or wronging any man by it.

I will not give a fatal draught to anyone if I am asked, nor will I suggest any such thing. Neither will I give a woman means to procure an abortion.

I will be chaste and religious in my life and in my practice.

I will not cut, even for the stone, but I will leave such procedures to the practitioners of that craft.

Whenever I go into a house, I will go to help the sick and never with the intention of doing harm or injury. I will not abuse my position to indulge in sexual contacts with the bodies of women or of men, whether they be freemen or slaves.

Whatever I see or hear, professionally or privately, which ought not to be divulged, I will keep secret and tell no one.
If, therefore, I observe this Oath and do not violate it, may I prosper both in my life and in my profession, earning good repute among all men for my time. If I transgress and forswear this oath, may my lot be otherwise."

Modern ethical codes

At first glance, the original oath of Hippocrates may appear to have little resemblance to modern versions and there may be aspects that would have no relevance to the practice of medicine and health care today. However, closer perusal shows that certain parts of the original oath have survived and still apply to health-care ethics.

Hippocrates swore to keep his patients from harm and injustice, never to give a 'fatal draught' or to make an incision but to work for the benefit of all sick people, not to abuse patients (whether they be slaves or free) and never to disclose any secrets confided in him. Today practitioners do not have to consider whether their patients are free or slaves and the suggestion of avoiding incisions cannot be reconciled with the increasing demand for surgery and the development of new techniques. Nonetheless, the parallels with the modern principles of health-care ethics – beneficence, non-maleficience, protection of the vulnerable and confidentiality (discussed in later chapters) – are there.

The survival of the Hippocratic Oath through history, and its treatment as a basis for modern medical and healthcare ethics, may have been attributed to its concordance with Christian ethics (Veatch 1997). It has been modernized, with sections altered or removed, but the underlying principle of a duty that the health-care practitioner has to patients, and the ways in which that duty should be respected and manifested, remains.

A significant development in modern ethics, from the Anglo-Saxon perspective, came from Thomas Percival, a physician. His foray into ethics emerged from a dispute between staff at the Manchester Infirmary, following a serious epidemic in 1789. Percival, who had been employed at the Infirmary, was asked by trustees to produce a document that would provide staff with guidance on how to conduct themselves professionally

(Veatch 1997). This document extended the basic essence of the Hippocratic Oath to include ethics as applied to working in institutions: good working relations with other professionals, manners and dignified behaviour (Veatch 1997). It can be said to have formed the basis for the principle of collegiality (discussed later).

In the aftermath of the Second World War, the World Medical Association (WMA) noted that standards of ethics in medicine and health care had been eroded. It was decided that a unifying international oath be developed and, in 1948, such an oath, the Declaration of Geneva, was adopted. It incorporated the basics of the Hippocratic Oath.

Declaration of Geneva (1948) (Physician's Oath)

At the time of being admitted as a member of the medical profession:

- I solemnly pledge myself to consecrate my life to the service of humanity;
- I will give to my teachers the respect and gratitude which is their due;
- I will practice my profession with conscience and dignity; the health of my patient will be my first consideration;
- I will maintain by all the means in my power, the honor and the noble traditions of the medical profession; my colleagues will be my brothers;
- I will not permit considerations of religion, nationality, race, party politics or social standing to intervene between my duty and my patient;
- I will maintain the utmost respect for human life from the time of conception, even under threat, I will not use my medical knowledge contrary to the laws of humanity;
- I make these promises solemnly, freely and upon my honor.

The following year, in response to a report about War Crimes committed by doctors under the Nazi regime, the WMA drafted a code of ethics that was appended to the Declaration of Geneva. This was adopted by the WMA as the International Code of Medical Ethics (1949). *See over*

International Code of Medical Ethics (WMA 1949)

Duties of Doctors in General

A doctor must always maintain the highest standards of professional conduct.
A doctor must practice his profession uninfluenced by motives of profit.
The following practices are deemed unethical:

    a. Any self advertisement except such as is expressly authorized by the national code of medical ethics;

    b. Collaborating in any form of medical service in which the doctor does not have professional independence;

    c. Receiving any money in connection with services rendered to a patient other than a proper professional fee, even with the knowledge of the patient.

Any act, or advice which could weaken physical or mental resistance of a human being may be used only in his interest.

A doctor is advised to use great caution in divulging discoveries or new techniques of treatment.

A doctor should certify or testify only to that which he has personally verified.

Duties of Doctors to the Sick

A doctor must always bear in mind the obligation of preserving human life from conception. Therapeutic abortion may only be performed if the conscience of the doctors and the national laws permit.

A doctor owes to his patients complete loyalty and all the resources of his science. Whenever an examination or treatment is beyond his capacity he should summon another doctor who has the necessary ability.

A doctor shall preserve absolute secrecy on all he knows about his patient because of the confidence entrusted in him.

A doctor must give emergency care as a humanitarian duty unless he is assured that others are willing and able to give such care.

Duties of Doctors to Each Other

A doctor ought to behave to his colleagues as he would have them behave to him.
A doctor must not entice patients from his colleagues.
A doctor must observe the principles of The Declaration of Geneva approved by the World Medical Association.

The codes of ethics of other healthcare professions incorporate relevant aspects of these codes.

MORALITY

"Moral philosophy is hard thought about right action."

(Socrates)

The origin and evolution of ethics show that ethics is grounded in morality. There is sometimes a tendency to use the terms ethics and morals interchangeably or to define ethics as a moral code. This may oversimplify the understanding of ethics, because morals are considered by many people to be guides to what is right and what is wrong. Those who are seeking answers to ethical problems may look to a moral code for guidance and expect a straightforward 'right/wrong' answer. But morality may be more than just a question of what is right and what is wrong, and will depend on an individual's interpretation of and degree of adherence to morals. At one end of the spectrum, hedonists may live without any regard to right or wrong. At the other end, strict moralists may have clear and very rigid ideas of what is right and what is wrong. The danger with such an approach is that it can precipitate extreme and even, what may be considered by many, bizarre behaviour.

The case of the late President Niyazov of Turkmenistan was an example of this. He published a moral code for the people of Turkmenistan in his Book of the Soul, the *Ruhnama* or *Ruhknama* (both spellings have been used). This was compulsory reading for all and graduation from schools and universities depended on knowledge of the *Ruhnama*. It is notable that physicians in Turkmenistan had to swear an oath to the President and not to Hippocrates. The foreword to the *Ruhnama* seemed acceptable and even admirable. It referred to maintenance of healthy living, cleanliness, intellectual rigour, integrity and good manners. It is hard to argue that any of these is bad for people or collectively for a nation. (It may be particularly pleasing for females to read that the President advocated that men liberally gift their womenfolk with gemstones and that they should never upset their wives or daughters.) However acceptable these words may have appeared, the fact that this moral code (coupled with other more bizarre decrees given below) was imposed on the people of Turkmenistan rendered it oppressive. When morality is forced on people and deviations from a rigorous moral code are punished, morals become laws. People living under such regimes follow the moral code for fear of retribution and not because they have considered and developed their own personal principles.

Some decrees of President Niyazov of Turkmenistan *(BBC News 2004a,b)*

- Opera and ballet music is forbidden.
- Long hair or beards for young men are forbidden.
- Car radios have been banned.
- Video monitors are required in all public places.
- All hospitals, except those in the capital, have been closed.
- Some calendar months have been named after the President and his mother.
- Passing an exam on the morals coded in the *Rukhmana* is a vital part of obtaining a driving licence.

Most people are not strict moralists or dictatorial in their beliefs. They have some basic principles to which they may adhere to a greater or lesser extent. People who are more devout in their religious beliefs may have a stronger set of morals that can help them to decide what is right and what is wrong. Yet, even with strong beliefs, there are times when the question of what is morally right or wrong can be difficult to answer.

Case study

Betty and John have been married for 5 years. They have three children under the age of the 3 years, the second pregnancy having produced twins. Betty has recently discovered that she is pregnant again, but this time the doctors have news that Betty has found disturbing. Ultrasound and serum screening tests have shown that the baby has anencephaly. This occurs when the upper part of the neural tube does not close as it should, resulting in the absence of a large part of the brain. If the baby is born alive, it will be deformed and would not be expected to live beyond a few days. The pregnancy and birth are not expected to pose any excessive risk to Betty but, after researching the subject and seeing pictures of anencephaly in live and stillborn babies, she is unsure of whether she wants to continue with the pregnancy.

Both Betty and John are religious and have always been strongly opposed to abortion. They believe that life is precious and that every baby should be given a chance to live regardless of whether there is an abnormality present.

Continued

However, Betty knows that this baby will not live. It has a very high chance of being stillborn and, even if it is alive when born, will not live beyond a few days. Betty is not sure whether she can face taking this pregnancy to term and she has three very young children to consider. For Betty and John the question of whether abortion was moral or not had always been answered with the underlying assumption that abortion was taking a life. They are left wondering whether the assumption is still valid in this case. The question for Betty and John is whether Betty should continue with the pregnancy (which, like any pregnancy, will not be without some, albeit minimal, risk) or whether she should terminate a life that she knows will not extend beyond a few days after birth and devote her time and energy to her existing children.

Morality is a complex web of factors based on beliefs and values. Beliefs and values themselves depend on a number of influences that include family background, schooling, religion, the impact of peers, and even the effects of hobbies and lifestyle.

With such a list of diverse influences, it is not surprising that morality can and does vary from individual to individual. Even siblings, who come from the same background and are likely to have had the same schooling and possibly religious teachings, can have a different set of morals. Peers, interests and hobbies will probably vary and these may have a significant impact on the development of moral values that can lead to very different lifestyle choices. An example of this is seen with the Clinton brothers. Bill Clinton was the President of the United States of America from 1993 to 2001. His half-brother, Roger, had problems with substance abuse from teenage years. He became a cocaine dealer and eventually spent 2 years in prison (Conley 2004).

In addition to the multifactorial influences that can shape morals and how they govern behaviour, it should be noted that morals are not static, but can, and often do, change with time. What a person may have once accepted as right may, years later, be treated as wrong. Conversely, practices that were once regarded as immoral may subsequently be considered morally acceptable. Views and opinions about what is moral may change as a person develops, encounters people with differing lifestyles and beliefs, and comes across situations that lead to a questioning of or a challenge to long-held moral principles. Sometimes these alterations may involve only subtle life changes, but they can lead to a significant change in moral outlook. Something as simple as changing dietary habits, from eating meat to becoming a vegetarian, can be based on the adoption of a new and strict set of morals about the mistreatment of animals. Conversely, what may appear to others to be a dramatic change in lifestyle may not involve any change in basic morals. A convert from Christianity to Islam may have retained the same set of morals based on religious views, but may have considered that the lifestyle practices of Islam adhere most closely to their set of morals.

Whether actions based on morals are grounded in reasoned judgements or are derived from intuition is still hotly debated. One famous theory about moral development is that of Kohlberg (1958) (referenced in Crain 1985), who based his studies on Piaget's theories of cognitive development. Kohlberg conducted a study of 72 boys in three age groups of 10, 13 and 16 years in which he presented them with a number of hypothetical situations and asked each boy how he thought the person in that given situation should respond and why. From the responses given by the children, Kohlberg theorized that there are three levels of moral development, each with two stages of reasoning. As a child's moral reasoning develops, its response moves progressively to a higher level and stage on Kohlberg's scale. One of the hypothetical situations used by Kohlberg is Heinz' dilemma, which has become a famous and often cited case study.

Heinz' dilemma

A woman was dying from cancer. Only one particular medication could save her life. This was a type of radium that had been discovered by a pharmacist who was selling the medication for ten times the price that it cost him to produce it. The husband of the sick woman, Heinz, did not have the money to buy the medication, so he went to all the people he knew to borrow money. He managed to get half of what the drug cost and took this to the pharmacist. He asked the pharmacist to sell the drug to him for half the price or to allow him to pay for the other half of the cost at a later date. The pharmacist refused to accept either offer. In desperation, Heinz broke into the pharmacy to steal the medication for his wife.

Should Heinz have stolen the medication?

The responses to Heinz' dilemma and the reasons for each response are categorized under Kohlberg's stages of moral reasoning (Table 1.1).

Table 1.1 Moral reasoning: Heinz' dilemma (adapted from Kohlberg et al 1983)		
Moral reasoning stage	**Response to dilemma**	**Reason for response**
Stage 1 – based on obedience	Heinz should not steal the medication	Because he will be punished and sent to prison
Stage 2 – based on self-interest	Heinz should steal the medication	Because it would make him happier to save his wife
Stage 3 – based on conformity	Heinz should steal the medication	Because it is what his wife expects him to do
Stage 4 – based on law/order	Heinz should not steal the medication	Because it is against the law
Stage 5 – based on human rights	Heinz should not steal the medication OR Heinz should steal the medication	Because the pharmacist has a right to receive payment for his discovery OR Because his wife has a right to live
Stage 6 – based on universal ethics	Heinz should not steal the medication OR Heinz should steal the medication	Because theft is an act of dishonesty and disrespect OR Because the right to life is greater than the right to payment for a discovery

A moral code in health care

Given the many possible influences on the shaping and development of morals and the fact that these influences can alter with time, it is not surprising that there is no universal moral code that has the answers to what is right and what is wrong in any given situation. Although such a broadly applicable moral code may be over-ambitious, could some semblance of a code be found if the perspective were narrowed to health care alone? In other words, are there specific moral principles that can be applied to health care at all times and that can provide a fundamental basis for an ethical code?

Four primary principles for health care have been outlined by Beauchamp & Childress (1994). They can be described as:

1. Practitioners should be fair to all patients.
2. Practitioners are obliged to perform duties to the best of their ability.
3. Practitioners should never inflict harm on anyone in health care.
4. Practitioners should encourage the maximum possible patient choice and decision.

These are sound principles; being fair, doing the best for patients, not hurting anyone and respecting patient choice would appear to have absolute and universal applicability. Yet, for each of these principles, there are situations that would render their application difficult, impractical or in conflict with another principles.

Being fair

An elderly woman presents with senile macular degeneration. She desperately wants help to have her sight restored. She is distraught and frightened. The practitioner will have to tell her that there is little that can be done to restore lost vision, but this is not what she wants to hear. Is it fair to distress such a patient by conveying to her the absolute truth: that she is likely to lose more of her sight? She needs to be prepared for this in time, but is it always advisable to tell the patient all the bad news at once, particularly if the patient presents in a particularly vulnerable state?

Performing duties to the very best of your abilities

This requires the practitioner to be aware of what standard of care and practice is the very best for him or her and to strive to meet this standard at all times. Yet every person will have good days and bad days, and there will be times when a practitioner is not feeling well or may be having personal problems that affect performance at work. The practitioner may still be a good practitioner but be unable at all times to perform to their own best standard.

Avoidance of harm

It is clear that a practitioner should never set out deliberately to harm a patient or to be involved in causing a patient unnecessary injury. What should be done about a patient who presents requesting referral for laser surgery? The refractive error and ocular health of this patient indicate that she is at a relatively low risk of harmful side-effects of this surgery. Nevertheless any surgical technique carries some risk of harm and it is questionable whether any such risk should be taken on a healthy eye for which surgery is not necessary. By referring the patient for this procedure, the practitioner could be deemed to be putting her in a potentially harmful situation. Yet, the patient is adamant that she wants this surgery and respect for the patient's decision dictates that she should be referred. Adhering to one of the moral principles may make it impossible to abide by another.

Respecting patients' decisions

A patient comes in for an annual check-up and the practitioner notices that the prescription has changed significantly – so significantly that the patient's vision is now below the legal limit permissible for driving. The patient refuses to change his prescription. Respecting the choice of the patient would potentially endanger the safety of the patient and others.

Just as there is no universal moral code, there is no principle in health care that is at all times applicable, and conflicts between principles can arise. This apparent inconsistency may be a little perplexing for those who are starting in healthcare practice and would prefer more rigid, less varying, regulations, rather like the law.

THE LAW

Laws are less flexible than morals because they regulate what is permissible and what is not. Unlike morals, which vary depending on the individual, laws have to be obeyed in the same way by all. Laws tell us what is right and what is wrong in accordance with what the government and judiciary decide. In order for a society to function in an ordered way, the law cannot be flexible and left to interpretation. This would clearly lead to confusion and potential anarchy.

Although there are strong links between ethics, morals and the law, and many laws have a basis in morality, there are also discrepancies and differences. Some actions are immoral and illegal, for example deliberately hurting or harming another person. There are acts that are both moral and legal, such as honest behaviour. However, laws and morals may sometimes come into conflict. An act that is legal may be considered, by some people, to be immoral. A good example of this is adultery. Conversely, an illegal act, such as assisted suicide, may not appear to be immoral if it is the wish of a loved one suffering from a painful and terminal disease. Laws may be related to ethics, but to rely solely on the law would make ethics too rigid. Laws are made for a society and are therefore general. They cannot take into account the many and diverse needs that arise within the remits of healthcare practice.

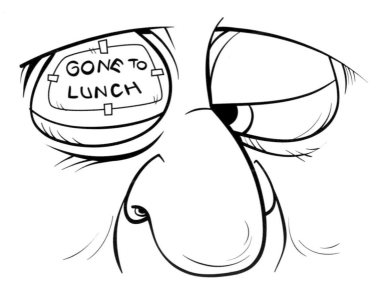

UNIVERSAL PRINCIPLES OF CHARACTER

Looking only to laws, rules or principles for developing a set of ethics can be very difficult because laws, rules and principles rely on actions: what should or should not be done. This is only one aspect of ethical development. The other is character: what we should strive to be in addition to what we should strive to do. Lennick & Kiel (2005) have identified four universal beliefs or principles of character that are cross-cultural: integrity, responsibility, compassion and forgiveness. A practitioner who develops these character traits will find that ethical practice and behaviour, both in the clinical situation and in personal life, will be a natural consequence.

"Rules cannot substitute for character."

(Lennick & Kiel 2005)

SUMMARY

Ethics have a basis in morality and some relationship to law, but in the practice of health care they cannot be as individual as personal moral beliefs or as rigid as the law. Ethics are general guidelines that practitioners are obliged to apply in practice in order to make balanced decisions. Their application may vary according to the judgement and personal principles of each practitioner, and may also alter with time and evolve with experience as a practitioner faces situations that require making decisions that may be challenging and difficult. Development of character is the best foundation for development of ethics in practice.

References

BBC News 2004a. Turkmen drivers face unusual test. BBC News 2 August 2004. Online. Available: http://news.bbc.co.uk/2/hi/asia-pacific/3528746.stm

BBC News 2004b. Turkmenistan bans recorded music (international version). BBC News 23 August 2005. Online. Available: http://news.bbc.co.uk/2/hi/asia-pacific/4177622.stm

Beauchamp T L, Childress J F 1994 Principles of biomedical ethics, 4th edn. Oxford University Press, New York

Chadwick J, Mann W N (trans) 1950 Hippocratic writings. Penguin Books, London

Conley D 2004 The pecking order: which siblings succeed and why, 1st edn. Pantheon, New York

Crain W C 1985 Kohlberg's stages of moral development. In: Theories of development. Prentice-Hall, New Jersey, pp 118–136

Declaration of Geneva 1948 Adopted by the General Assembly of the World Medical Association, Geneva, Switzerland, September 1948. Online. Available: http://www.cirp.org/library/ethics/geneva/

Kohlberg L, Levine C, Hewer A 1983 Moral stages: a current formulation and a response to critics. Karger, Basel

Lennick D, Kiel F 2005 Moral intelligence: enhancing business performance and leadership success. Wharton School Publishing, Philadelphia

Re A (Children) Court of Appeal (Civil Division) [2000] The Times 10 Oct 2000, The Independent 3 Oct 2000, 150 NLJ 1453

Re Wyatt (a child) (medical treatment: parents' consent), Family Division [2004] EWHC 2247 (Fam); 84 BMLR 206, 7 Oct 2004

Re Wyatt Family Division [2006] EWHC 319 (Fam), 2 FLR 111, 23 Feb 2006

Veatch R M 1997 Medical ethics: an introduction in medical ethics, 2nd edn. Jones & Bartlett, Sudbury, MA, pp 1–29

World Medical Association 1949 International code of medical ethics. World Medical Association Bulletin 1(3):109, 111

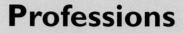

Professions

"Professions are conspiracies against the laity."
(George Bernard Shaw, preface to *The Doctor's Dilemma*)

THE HISTORY AND DEVELOPMENT OF PROFESSIONS

It is difficult to ascertain when the concept of a profession began. In terms of health care, the Hippocratic Oath was an early attempt to establish medicine as a profession because, in Hippocrates' time, cures could be dispensed by anyone for any price they wished to charge. Not surprisingly, this lack of prohibition led to a variety of spiritualists as well as fraudsters who offered treatments for all sorts of illnesses and ailments. Consultations with Oracles, particularly the one at Delphi dedicated to Apollo (father of Asclepius, the god of healing), were also not uncommon. By introducing an oath that served as a code of practice, Hippocrates aimed to distinguish trained practitioners of medicine from those who merely dispensed treatment, potions and advice.

One of the earliest English definitions for a profession, as accepted in common usage, can be found in the dictionary of Samuel Johnson from 1756. According to Dr Johnson, it is a 'calling; vocation; known employment … particularly used of divinity, physick and law' (Johnson 1756). This confirmed the writings of the famous genealogist Gregory King, who studied the demographics and wealth of England and Wales in the late 17th century. He placed bureaucrats ('persons in offices'), lawyers, clergymen and 'persons in science and liberal arts' (this included medical practitioners and teachers) in the category of professions (Arkell 2006).

The definition of professions then was dependent on the groups that were perceived to fit into a class that was established in order to distinguish a separate group between the aristocracy and tradesmen (O'Day 2000). They were a group that were educated and therefore did not have to work manually, but not sufficiently wealthy to live without having to earn a salary. Although there was little reference to ethics, professional groups provided services that in some way offered help and, particularly with the inclusion of clergy, formed a link between profession and vocation.

THE MEANING OF A PROFESSION TODAY

The modern usage of the term 'professional' is now employed in a far wider context than in the past, from describing individuals who have qualifications, specialist training and expertise to those who perform or engage in a specific activity for which they are paid. Hence, we find that a doctor, who is highly educated and qualified, is a professional. A football player who plays football for a living can also be referred to as a professional sportsperson. Yet there is a great deal of difference between the doctor and the football player. Doctors have had to undergo years of study and to complete various stages of training to obtain a qualification. After qualifying, they need to continue their training and education throughout their life in practice. Football players may have certain sporting abilities and skills but these have not required years of study. Football players do not need to possess any formal qualifications. They must keep training to maintain their sporting abilities and physical strength, but are not expected or required to advance knowledge or learning.

According to the Oxford English Dictionary (1989) definition, a profession is defined as an 'occupation/vocation' with 'some professed knowledge of some department of learning or science'. This definition is easy to apply to the doctor, the lawyer, the optometrist or the teacher. It is clearly inapplicable to the football player or indeed to any sportsperson. It may not even appear to be quite so clear for the electrician, the mechanic or the plumber. Whether or not these are classed as professions depends on how 'learning' is defined. If learning is taken as the acquisition of knowledge through a traditional academic route, then, according to the Oxford Dictionary, these occupations are not categorized as professions. Indeed, the occupations in which plumbers, electricians and mechanics engage are not generally considered to be professions but are referred to as trades.

The distinction between professions and other occupations

There are a number of special characteristics that distinguish a profession from a trade or any other occupation. Jones (2003) provided six main criteria that can be used to characterize a group as a profession:

- that there is a well defined body of knowledge that is controlled by the members of the group;
- that there is no market-based competition for the services of the group;
- that the group enjoys autonomy or self-regulation over working conditions;
- that the group possesses a code of ethics;
- that members of the group have altruistic motives with a greater emphasis placed on performance achieved than money earned;
- that there is a substantial training, regulated and controlled by the group.

Jones (2003) focused on the medical profession, and the same criteria, again with the emphasis on medical professionals, have been given by Hope et al (2003), based on the work of Bayles (1988). The consistency in certain of these criteria is seen when comparing the meaning of profession applied to the law and accountancy. Empson (2007), who has defined professionalism in law, accountancy and service consulting firms, cites the aspects of training, accreditation, self-regulation and an ethical code as requisites for a profession. Empson (2007), however, also raises the prospect of higher social status and wealth associated with the recognition of a professional. This contrasts sharply with the criteria of altruism (Jones 2003) or commitment to serve the public (Hope et al 2003) that distinguish the medical/healthcare professions from business and the law.

There is no doubt that being a professional means belonging to an organization or body that regulates, monitors and sets guidelines for conduct. This body is recognized by law and it gives accreditation to the educational courses that individuals have to undergo and complete to a certain standard in order to belong to the profession. Completion of such a course results in a qualification, which is

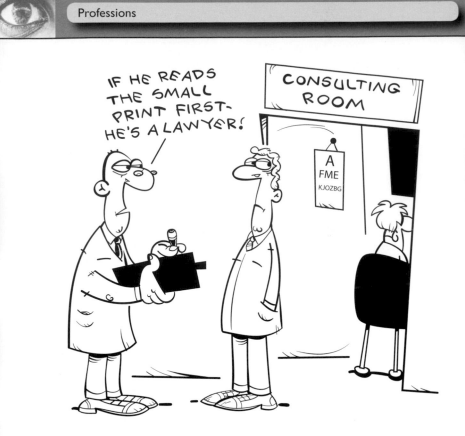

another distinctive feature of a profession. Professionals should continue to expand their knowledge and improve their skills by attending educational seminars, conferences and training courses that provide updates on new advances. Every profession has a number of journals in which the latest findings in that particular discipline are published. Professionals have a recognized status in society, a certain degree of prestige and an income that is often higher than that earned by non-professionals (although the distinction based on earnings is becoming more blurred). Doctors, lawyers, optometrists and veterinary surgeons, amongst others, clearly fit the criteria listed by Jones (2003), and there is a societal recognition that these are professions. Yet, what Jones (2003) proposes may not be acceptable to all. Nursing, for example, would not qualify as a profession according to Jones' characterization because nursing is not practised independently, i.e. nurses generally report to another professional group, usually to doctors.

There are a number of occupations that may be classed as professional by society yet they do not meet the criteria expected of the medical or healthcare practitioner. Good examples of these are journalism, politics or management. Journalists are a well defined group and are expected to meet certain standards, but these standards are not a code of ethics. Whilst there are degrees in journalism, it is possible to become a journalist via a number of other routes. Managers may meet all of the listed criteria: they may have specific managerial qualifications, such as an MBA, belong to a professional body, and continue to update their knowledge from continuing education and journals. Yet the term 'manager' can also be used for anyone who manages a shop or office and has no qualifications or special skills in any discipline. Thus, not all managers are professionals. Politicians are representatives of the community. They have a very important status in society and yet they are not professionals, at least not with regard to politics. They are not a separate group that is defined by a specific discipline or qualification. There is a ministerial code that outlines acceptable practice, but it is not a code of ethics. Empson (2007) points out that for some groups, such as investment bankers, who enjoy a very high social status and associated wealth, there is a perception that this is a professional group, even though no specific qualification is required and no ethical code exists. Such a perception is based on a looser interpretation of professionalism than is used in medicine and the healthcare professions.

As a discipline evolves and its members expand their training and practice, a non-professional occupation can take on the characteristics of a profession or can deem itself to be a profession. This can lead to further confusion in the definition of a profession. According to the Professional Associations Research Network (PARN: http://www.parn.org.uk) there are around 400 professional associations in the UK. These include the traditional professions as well as new and emerging specialist groups that consider themselves to be professionals. Not all of these groups meet the criteria outlined for a profession. For example, the Royal Society for the Promotion of Health, which is listed as a professional association under PARN, is a charity. It runs diploma courses on topics that include nutrition, health and safety, pest control and meat inspection. Membership requires a degree in a health-related field or a diploma obtained from the Royal Society for the Promotion of Health. This illustrates the ease with which a group or body can call itself a professional association. A distinction needs to be made between an association such as the Royal Society for the Promotion of Health and a truly professional body, membership of which requires a particular qualification obtained to a certain standard. The confusion largely arises because there is no regulation that requires a group to meet strict criteria before it can use the word professional to describe its members.

The one distinguishing feature that marks a profession from other occupations or trades is the obligation to practise ethically. Every professional body, if it is truly a professional body, should have a code of ethics. The obligation to practise ethically is reflected in societal expectations on professionals to be ethical and to behave in a responsible, trustworthy and respectable way. Expectations of behaviour extend beyond working time. Optometrists do not cease to be optometrists when they leave the consulting room. Even when not actively practising, an optometrist remains a professional and his or her behaviour is judged according to the standards that society expects of a professional.

> ### Teacher jailed
>
> In May 2004 a group of British men were jailed for organizing violence between rival club football fans. The only member of the group whose occupation was mentioned, and who was singled out by the media, was a high school teacher. He was not the most serious offender of the group. The fact that this man was a professional made his association with acts of hooliganism more shocking to society than the involvement of the others in the group. On his release, the General Teaching Council barred him from ever teaching again. (BBC News 24 2004a,b)

MOTIVES AND THE CHOICE OF PROFESSION

The way in which a practitioner approaches ethics in practice can be linked to the reasons why he or she has chosen that particular profession. There are three main motivating reasons that an individual may choose to enter a healthcare profession such as optometry. The choice may be based on one or more of these:

- idealistic motives
- materialistic motives
- realistic motives.

Idealistic motives are based on wanting to help people and to serve society. An idealistic professional will be concerned primarily with serving the needs of others. The admirable traits of idealistic professionals are that they are caring and concerned practitioners who have the highest standards of patient care. The risk with the idealistic practitioner is that he or she may expect the same exacting standards of other practitioners. Such a practitioner may even place too many demands on him or herself and find that meeting such high ethical standards is sometimes very hard. This may detract from enjoyment of professional practice.

People who enter optometry with materialistic motives may be attracted principally to the status, earnings and subsequent financial security that such a profession can offer. This is not necessarily a bad motive. A substantial salary and status will enable a person to provide a higher standard of living for their family. The materialistically motivated practitioner may have a number of other interests, some of which may be beneficial to society and he or she may be able to contribute some earnings to these causes. The materialistic practitioner will also need to have a regard to ethical practice for there is a danger of substandard care if the desire for a high salary becomes the sole purpose for practice. Creating profit at the expense of patient care can lead to an erosion of ethical standards.

The realistic practitioner chooses a healthcare profession such as optometry because it offers a reasonable salary and flexible, family-friendly hours. In the past this may have been the prime motivating factor for women to choose optometry. Increasingly, these reasons are becoming more important for both sexes as more men want to be actively involved in parenting and family life. The realistically motivated practitioner needs to watch that the balance of work and family is such that neither suffers and that demands of family life do not encroach on standards of practice.

Case study

Jack, Mary and John graduated as optometrists in the same year. Each was an able and intelligent student and each had clearly defined ambitions. Jack chose to work in a hospital in the deprived areas of the inner city dealing with people with physical disabilities and low vision problems. He is motivated to help members of society who have significant sight impairments and limited access to care.

Continued

Mary chose optometry because she was attracted by the money that can be earned by optometrists. She works for a multiple practice where she is paid a substantial salary. She has a number of other interests and commitments. The money she earns in optometry allows her to continue to be involved in these activities. She is also actively involved in the profession, sits on a number of committees, and contributes to the development and growth of optometry and its links with other healthcare professions.

John chose optometry because he wanted to have a family and to be actively involved in parenting. He arranges his working hours so that he can collect his children from school twice a week and share equally in the role of parenting with his wife.

Each of these practitioners practises ethically but their motives, goals, values and judgements are quite different.

A MEASURE OF SUCCESS

What does it mean to be a success? The definition of success, and particularly how a practitioner measures his or her professional success, is linked to motives for entering the chosen profession.

An idealistically motivated optometrist may consider that success is measured by the number of patients who are helped with their vision, sight or refractive problems. The materialistically motivated practitioner will link success to the profits made and status attained. The realistically motivated practitioner will measure success by looking at how well the work/life balance has been achieved.

Society, in general, tends to measure success by material wealth, fame and, more recently, recognition and celebrity status. Sometimes this leads to the question of what such measures of success have achieved for society. The scientist who becomes famous by making a new discovery that could lead to curing of a certain disease has succeeded in using their talents to benefit the world. The rich businessman who owns a chain of retail stores, selling trendy clothing made in sweat shops in the third world that exploit child labour, may consider himself to be successful. If his sole aim is to accumulate wealth, he is indeed a success. Yet, when personal goals are predicated on the degradation and exploitation of others, the value of such success is questionable. More vague are the determinants of success of celebrities who become household names by appearing on reality programmes in which they do little else than talk with other participants. The value of these interactions to society is not clear. Critics of reality programmes have even considered that these participants are being denigrated and victimized, a view that clearly contradicts any reference to success.

If success is measured by recognition and wealth, individuals who are teachers, scientists and healthcare practitioners would appear to be less successful than those who are famous actors, entertainers, sportspersons and reality show participants. However, if recognition of the individual is transposed to recognition of the value of the group or profession to which he or she belongs, the trends are reversed. There is greater recognition, by society, of the value of teaching and medicine than of entertainment. It should also be noted that recognition and value can be transient and do alter with time.

Exercise 1

Name five famous people who are still alive from each of the following categories:

(a) actors
(b) sportspersons
(c) politicians
(d) scientists
(e) teachers/philosophers

For most people the exercise becomes harder with progression from (a) to (e). More actors, sporting personalities and politicians, rather than scientists and teachers, are given media coverage. They are therefore more likely to be recognized and remembered.

Exercise 2

Name five famous people who are no longer alive from each of the following categories:

(a) actors
(b) sportspersons
(c) politicians
(d) scientists
(e) teachers/philosophers

If the question is altered to name five people from each category who are no longer alive, the ease of naming starts to reverse. It becomes easier to name famous scientists and teachers from the past than it does sporting heroes and actors. This is even more evident when the question goes further back in history. How many famous actors who lived between the 15th and 19th centuries are known today? Compare this with the number of famous scientists from the same period. As one goes back to ancient history, the number of famous teachers/philosophers who can be named increases. Sporting heroes and entertainers from the ancient world are relatively unknown (except perhaps to classics scholars). Those who have left their mark on society will be remembered for longer, even if they are not as well known in their lifetime. Those who are famous because they provide entertainment, be it through sports or other forms, are forgotten relatively quickly. This is because their success lasts as long as they are in the public eye. Little is left that can impact on or be valued by future generations. If we measure success by lasting recognition, those who provide the greatest benefit to or have the greatest impact on society are the most successful.

Personal success depends on the individual, their goals and their achievements. In optometry, as in other healthcare professions, these goals will involve the health provision aspect as well as the business side of practice. In terms of success there will be a balance between patient care and interests and the requirement to make money. This will be influenced by career choice motives and will also depend on practice type and size. In a large chain practice there may be more emphasis placed on the financial aspect than in a small private practice or hospital-based clinic. Ethics need not be compromised by a greater prominence given to the business side of practice. However, depending on the type of practice, there may also be a different emphasis on the various ethical principles. For example, the ethics of team working and collegiality may have more relevance in a hospital clinic than in a private practice with a single practitioner. Advertising the price of spectacles or vision aids may be ethical for a multiple chain of practices but may not be acceptable for an optometrist working in a hospital. This is because marketing and advertising are an essential part of the business aspect of a multi-chain practice. Marketing has less relevance in a public service institution such as a hospital. In accordance with the variety of practice types, the application of ethics to optometric as well as other healthcare practice can take many forms.

Each of these forms should be appropriate to the practice and each should comply with the professional code.

THE FUTURE OF PROFESSIONS

The rapid growth in the number of professional associations and the concomitant blurring of distinction between traditional professions and newly emerging occupations that also claim professional status has led to an increasingly liberal use of the term professional.[1] This is evident from the recent definition of a profession provided by Cheetham & Chivers (2005):

> *"an occupation based upon specialised study, training or experience, the purpose of which is to apply skilled service or advice to others, or to provide technical, managerial or administrative services to, or within, organisations in return for a fee or salary."*

According to this definition, a specialist cleaner with some experience and skill could claim professional status, but the university research academic, whose specialist subject is philosophy, may not qualify (depending on the definition of 'skilled service'). The philosopher works within an organization but researching philosophy is neither a technical, managerial nor administrative service.

Cheetham and Chivers' definition may be aimed at encompassing all groups that wish to be considered as professional yet it can actually exclude the highly educated in favour of those with no education. It is contrary to most definitions that consider specialized education and training as a vital characteristic of a profession. Moreover, it lacks any mention of ethics. An all-inclusive definition such as this may serve to confound rather than to crystallize and fortify a set of specific criteria for a profession. Beauchamp & Childress (2001) have noted the need for a more limited and better controlled definition of a profession, and point out that the blurring of boundaries between traditional professions and occupations has led to the term *learned professional*, to distinguish highly

---

[1]Broad meanings of 'profession' have been offered in a number of sociological articles and essays for decades. There are too many to cite and some are poorly considered and completely misrepresent the meaning of a profession. An example of one of these is the definition of Parsons (cited in Beauchamp & Childress 2001, p 6): 'a cluster of occupational roles … in which incumbents perform certain functions valued in the society and by these activities, typically earn a living at a full-time job'.

educated professionals from those who earn a living by engaging in an occupation.

Campbell (1988) outlined the three approaches to defining professions:

- 'trait' – based on the traits of established professions;
- 'power' – based on the model for medicine; and
- 'functionalist' – based on social necessity and usefulness.

The difficulty with the first approach is the ever-changing notion of what represents an established profession. The second approach, using medicine as a model for all professions, may cause confusion in professions beyond the boundaries of health care. Although altruistic motives that concern serving the best interests of patients are fine for the healthcare practitioner, they cannot be applied to the criminal lawyer defending a client who informs the lawyer that he has indeed committed the murder but intends to plead not guilty. The third, functionalist, approach based on usefulness to society opens the gates to any occupational group that is well organized (Campbell 1988) and can be deemed to be of value. (Footballers could feasibly qualify, if the sport is seen as providing a useful social function.)

Perhaps the time has come to return to the historical meaning of profession, particularly in health care, when the term had some sort of link to vocation. The word vocation comes from the Latin *vocare*, which means 'to call'. Profession is derived from *professio*, which means 'to avow publicly'. The two are not remotely different. If to be a professional means that a period of extensive education and training is required, if it means providing a service for more than mere remuneration and a commitment to work to the best possible personal standard, the public avowal is indeed an answer to a call. The link between the vocation and profession is evident. The role of ethics in modern professional practice reinforces this link.

It is notable that the Royal College of Physicians has recently reassessed the meaning of profession and produced a definition and description of medical professionalism. The description (shown below) refers to medicine as a vocation. It also includes a commitment to two of the four universal principles of character: integrity and compassion, identified by Lennick & Kiel (2005) (described in Chapter 1). A third principle of character, responsibility, is contained within the commitment to 'continuous improvement' and 'excellence'.

Royal College of Physicians' description of medical professionalism

"*Medicine is a vocation in which a doctor's knowledge, clinical skills, and judgment are put in the service of protecting and restoring human wellbeing. This purpose is realised through a partnership between patient and doctor, one based on mutual respect, individual responsibility, and appropriate accountability.*

In their day-to-day practice, doctors are committed to:

- *integrity*
- *compassion*
- *altruism*
- *continuous improvement*
- *excellence*
- *working in partnership with members of the wider health-care team.*

These values, which underpin the science and practice of medicine, form the basis for a moral contract between the medical profession and society. Each party has a duty to work to strengthen the system of health care on which our collective human dignity depends."

(cited in Horton et al 2007)

SUMMARY

The definition of profession has altered over centuries and continues to be poorly defined, largely because of the many and sometimes contradictory definitions that exist. With respect to medicine and health care, the feature that distinguishes these as professions rather than occupations is the requirement for ethics.

References

Arkell T 2006 Illuminations and distortions: Gregory King's Scheme for the year 1688 and the social structure of later Stuart England. Economic History Review LIX 1:32–69

Bayles M D 1988 The professions. In: Callahan J C (ed.) Ethical issues in professional life. Oxford University Press, New York, pp 27–30

BBC News 24 2004. Hooligans jailed over fight plot. BBC News 24 7 May 2004. Online. Available: http://news.bbc.co.uk/1/hi/uk/3693885.stm

BBC News 24 2004. Teacher banned after hooliganism. BBC News 24 7 July 2004. Online. Available: http://news.bbc.co.uk/1/hi/england/hampshire/5158970.stm

Beauchamp T L, Childress J F 2001 Principles of biomedical ethics, 5th edn. Oxford University Press, New York

Campbell A 1988 Profession and vocation. In: Fairburn G & Fairburn S (eds) Ethical issues in caring. Avebury Gower, Aldershot, pp 1–9

Cheetham G, Chivers G 2005 Professions, competence and informal learning. Edward Elgar, Cheltenham

Empson L 2007 Profession. In: Clegg S R & Bailey J R (eds) International encylcopedia of organization studies. Sage, Thousand Oaks. Online. Available: http://www.sbs.ox.ac.uk/ccc/Profession.htm

Hope T, Savulescu J, Hendrick J 2003 Medical ethics and law. Churchill Livingstone, Edinburgh pp 51–59

Horton R, Gilmore I, Dickson N, Dewer S, Shepherd S 2007 Do doctors have a future? Lancet 369:1405–1406

Johnson S 1756 Dictionary of the English language. British Library shelf-mark 1560/1901

Jones I R 2003 Health professions. In: Scambler G (ed.) Sociology as applied to medicine, 5th edn. Saunders, Edinburgh, pp 235–247

Lennick D, Kiel F 2005 Moral intelligence: enhancing business performance and leadership success. Wharton School Publishing, Philadelphia

O'Day R 2000 The professions in early modern England 1450–1800. Longman Higher Education, Harlow

Oxford English Dictionary, 2nd edn 1989 Oxford University Press, Oxford. Online. Available: http://dictionary.oed.com/cgi/entry/50189444?single=1&query_type=word&queryword=profession&first=1&max_to_show=10

Shaw G B 1911 The doctor's dilemma. Penguin, New York

The optometric code of ethics and basic ethical concepts

Optometry is a profession, the status and recognition of which varies from country to country. Unlike medical graduates who are universally recognized as doctors dealing with all general and/or specific aspects of health care, the understanding of what is an optometrist is not as well defined. Setting aside the countries where little or even no qualification is needed to open a shop in which the prescription and sale of spectacles takes place, the qualification of optometry graduates can range from a 3-year undergraduate degree with a year in clinical placement to a graduate programme from which students qualify as Doctors of Optometry.

OPTOMETRIC CODE OF ETHICS

The profession has, as every profession is required to have, a code of ethics. Like the status of the profession, the codes also vary from a single sentence, as applied to optometry in the United Kingdom, to the longer versions from the American and Australian optometric associations.

In the United Kingdom, the College of Optometrists (2007) has produced a Code of Ethics and Guidelines for Professional Conduct, which states:

Code of Ethics of the American Optometric Association

"It shall be the Ideal, the Resolve and the Duty of the Members of the American Optometric Association:

TO KEEP the visual welfare of the patient uppermost at all times;

TO PROMOTE in every possible way, in collaboration with this Association, better care of the visual needs of mankind;

TO ENHANCE continuously their educational and technical proficiency to the end that their patients shall receive the benefits of all acknowledged improvements in visual care;

TO SEE that no person shall lack for visual care, regardless of financial status;

TO ADVISE the patient whenever consultation with an optometric colleague or reference for other professional care seems advisable;

TO HOLD in professional confidence all information concerning a patient and to use such data only for the benefit of the patient;

TO CONDUCT themselves as exemplary citizens;

TO MAINTAIN their offices and their practices in keeping with professional standards;

TO PROMOTE and maintain cordial and unselfish relationships with members of their own profession and of other professions for the exchange of information to the advantage of mankind."

Adopted by the AOA House of Delegates as Substantive Motion 1 of 1944 (cited by Bailey & Heitman 2000).

The Code of Ethics of the Optometrists Association Australia is very similar to that of its US counterpart.

"An optometrist shall always place the welfare of the patient before all other considerations, and shall behave in a proper manner towards professional colleagues and shall not bring them or the profession into disrepute"

This relatively simple and basic form of code, compared with the more specific American and Australian codes, leaves more to interpretation. For example, the UK code makes no specific mention of exemplary behaviour as a citizen (which includes life beyond clinical practice). However, optometrists in the United Kingdom are asked not to behave in a way that could discredit the profession, and this encompasses conduct outside practice.

Accompanying the code of ethics are ten principles that support and expand the code, providing more specific guidance.

Guiding principles

"1. The practitioner should always have as his prime concern the welfare and safety of both patient and the public."

This appears to be obvious. Clearly an optometrist should be concerned with welfare of his or her patients. However, the principle describes more than this. It asks that the practitioner consider not only the ocular health and welfare of the patient but also patient safety. It is not sufficient to conduct a thorough examination and to treat patients in the best possible manner, if the prescription provided is, through mistake or carelessness, in error. A wrong prescription could lead to an accident. Injecting a mydriatic in an eye without explaining to the patient the consequences of a dilated pupil could result in more than just discomfort from excess light reaching retina. If the patient drives home, with temporarily impaired vision, this could cause a road accident that may also involve injury to another member of the public. The principle extends to cover not only those who are patients at the practice, but also to anyone who may be affected by what the optometrist prescribes and/or how he or she practises.

"2. The practitioner should ensure that he is adequately covered by public and products liability insurance which includes professional indemnity cover."

Insurance is necessary in most aspects of life: we insure our homes, our cars and even ourselves. So it is not surprising that insurance is an important part of professional life. Indeed, professional insurance has now become a legal requirement for registration with the General Optical Council (GOC) (section 10A The Opticians Act 1989 (Amendment) Order 2005). The legislation states that a practitioner must have 'adequate and appropriate insurance', and evidence of this must be provided to the GOC. The legislation gives the GOC the authority to decide what is 'adequate and appropriate'.

Insurance as a practitioner should not be considered to be solely for the safety of patients but also for the protection of the practitioner. Present trends in health care show a move to safeguarding patients' interests, and even the very best and most ethical practitioners may find themselves in a position of having to defend their practice methods. Take the situation of a practitioner who has good reason to dilate a patient's eyes and has found no contraindications to so doing after a thorough examination and case history. The angles are wide, there is no family or general history of glaucoma. The patient is fully informed and consents to the dilation. A few hours later, in spite of all efforts taken to check that risks are minimal, the patient has an attack of glaucoma and, despite having granted consent, the patient decides to take legal action. With thorough patient records, including one showing that consent was granted, the practitioner has a stronger chance of being cleared. However, legal representation and insurance cover will be required.

The practitioner is not the only part of the practice that needs insurance. Premises should also be insured. If a patient trips over in a practice and is hurt, the owner of the practice, usually the practitioner, could be liable. This liability could extend to persons who are not patients. For example, a tradesperson who may be hired for practice refurbishment may sustain an injury and may also, depending on causation, have a case against the owner of the premises. Insurance is needed to underwrite any expenses that may arise from such incidents. It is also prudent to insure the contents of the practice; equipment, frames, contact lenses and other optical devices that may be on the premises are costly items that need to be protected with some form of contents cover.

"3. The honour and dignity of the profession shall be upheld at all times and no activity shall be engaged in which might bring the profession into disrepute."

This principle is a reminder that a professional is a professional both during and outside working hours and that society expects a certain standard of behaviour from professionals. This includes dressing respectfully and behaving in a professional manner whilst at work, but it also means not engaging in activities, outside working life, that may be deemed to be disreputable. There is nothing alarming about an optometrist having a few drinks in a pub with some friends. However, if the evening ends in a brawl with police attendance and media interest, the greatest attention will be focused on the optometrist and any other professional who may have been involved.

The extent to which the behaviour of professionals outside working life can be scrutinized has been highlighted by a recent case of a teacher who stood as a candidate for the British National Party (BNP) and incited the wrath of a teachers' union (BBC News 2006). The argument that the BNP is a legitimate party and that the teacher had not broken any laws was insufficient to deter those who believed that belonging to such a party was inconsistent with professional conduct. The fact that professional conduct, and indeed what exactly is meant by being a professional, has no strict definition allows subjective interpretations to enter into decisions. Subjective interpretations are based on societal expectations. In some cases these are clear: a judge downloading child pornography (Jones 2004) or a teacher involved in hooliganism (BBC News 2004) clearly demonstrates disreputable behaviour that casts a slur on their professional status. The situation is less clear when a professional becomes inadvertently involved in an incident that is immediately seized upon by the media.

The solicitor in a kebab shop

In 2003, David Messenger was arrested in a kebab shop in Scarborough and charged with being drunk and disorderly and obstructing the police. Mr Messenger denied all allegations and claimed that he had gone to investigate a dispute in the kitchen of the shop, the owner of which was a client of Mr Messenger's. The police alleged that Mr Messenger was drunk, wilfully obstructed them and caused damage to a police cell alarm button. Mr Messenger asserted that he was not drunk, he had consumed about four beers in as many hours, he had intervened in the matter to help, and he had merely questioned the cause of his arrest (the legal right of every citizen). Both versions appear quite plausible. The Magistrates Court at Selby ruled in favour of the police. Such a matter is unlikely to have been reported in the press, given that no damage to property or injury to any person was sustained, yet Mr Messenger's case was broadcast in the media because he was a solicitor and a Deputy District Judge. The comments by the magistrate (Dr M Jones) give cause for reflection:

> "You don't need me to tell you that you have not only let yourself down but your profession. Any punishment we give you will be minor compared to the loss of your standing in the community."

(BBC News 2003a,b)

"4. The practitioner shall at all times have due regard to the laws and regulations applicable and maintain a high standard of professional conduct. Acts or omissions that might impair confidence in the profession should be avoided."

All practitioners need to keep themselves informed of laws and changes to laws and regulations that apply to professional practice. Ignorance of the law is not an acceptable excuse for breaking it. Similarly it is incumbent on the practitioner to review and keep abreast of statements, codes and standards published by the professional body. Practitioners should not rely on the professional body to act as a continual source of reminder notices about recent changes to standards or regulations.

In addition to the codes and standards published by the College of Optometrists, there are other aspects of professional life that may extend beyond what is covered by the College. Optometric practice can involve employment of others, buying and selling of premises, and purchasing of products. These aspects of practice management may require basic knowledge of employment, consumer and business law. A grievance claim by an employee or a dispute with a person to whom a practice is sold may have nothing to do with patient care; however, it can reflect negatively on the practitioner against whom a claim is made and this may have an impact on how that practitioner is regarded as a professional.

"5. Information relating to the health or welfare of any patient or person should be respected and remain confidential between practitioner and patient or person, unless disclosure is specifically permitted by such patient or person or by law."

Confidentiality is not only an ethical expectation but also a legal obligation. It dates back to the Hippocratic Oath and, since then, has always been an important aspect of health care that must be maintained and respected. How it is applied will vary depending on the practice. In a single practitioner practice, there will be no need for anyone else to see patient case history and examination results. In a larger practice, where more than one optometrist may see a patient, the patient data must be available to every practitioner who is treating that particular patient. Even in that situation, if a patient tells a practitioner something confidential that does not relate to vision or ocular care, and which does not need to be recorded, the practitioner should respect and keep this information in confidence. If patient data are being used for other purposes, such as research, the patient must give consent before the data can be used and the data should be kept confidential to the researcher(s). Consent can be given only once the patient is fully informed about the project and the consequences of data usage. There are a number of legal reasons that require disclosure of confidential information. These are outlined in Chapter 7 on confidentiality.

> "6. The practitioner should keep abreast of the progress of scientific and other relevant knowledge pertinent to the profession, seek to develop his professional competence and maintain a high standard of professional expertise relative to his sphere of activity."

Education does not end after graduation or after the pre-registration examinations. Scientific and technological as well as legal and ethical advances continue to be made. Healthcare practitioners are obliged to keep abreast of the latest developments and changes that may impact on professional practice. This will not only assist in professional development but will also enhance the practitioner's reputation with patients. For example, it could be an awkward experience for a practitioner to have a patient ask about the latest development in glaucoma treatment reported in the newspapers and yet to know nothing about this. The chances are that, if it has reached the popular press, it would most certainly have been published in some journal or professional magazine. If a practitioner is specializing in a particular area of optometry, there is an even greater need to keep up with latest developments in that specialist area. Specialization may require more than expert knowledge and learning the techniques relevant to that area. It may also involve investing in the latest equipment.

> "7. The practitioner should not agree to practise under any conditions of service which would prevent or impede his professional integrity, nor impose such conditions on other members of the profession."

Professional practice has no place for behaviour that may result in undermining the practitioner's professional and/or personal integrity. A practice manager, who is not qualified in optometry, may decide that 10 minutes is sufficient time to conduct examinations on all patients and that old and malfunctioning equipment should not be replaced. Such rigid working conditions would result in the optometrist being unable to conduct proper examinations. Inadequate examination can lead to an incorrect prescription or misdiagnosis of an underlying condition. Poorly functioning equipment at best provides no useful information and at worst may cause an injury. What may appear to the practice manager to be an efficient management model for maximizing income generation can result in an impedance to professional practice, and practitioners should not agree to work under such conditions. Time may be money, but not at the expense of patient care and practitioner integrity.

"8. Practitioners should co-operate with professional colleagues and members of other professions to the benefit of patients and the public."

Optometrists need to work with other optometrists as well as with other healthcare professionals. In many cases a patient may require a referral or a multi-team approach. Co-management of patient care is becoming ever more popular because it benefits patients as well as practitioners. Competing rather than co-operating with other professionals is counterproductive. Mutual respect for the skills and expertise of all members of a healthcare team generates trust and instils confidence in patients. Developing and nurturing relationships within and beyond optometry is therefore vital for strengthening and expanding the profession.

"9. No practitioner should criticise or cast doubts on the integrity of other professional colleagues except when absolute candour is required in the furnishing of evidence in legal or disciplinary proceedings, or if the practitioner considers that patients' welfare is being placed at risk through the actions of a professional colleague."

Unwarranted criticism of an optometric colleague means discrediting a member of the profession. When a practitioner discredits a member of his or her own profession, he or she *de facto* discredits him or herself. An optometrist who behaves in a manner that is unprofessional should be reminded in private about their conduct. In cases where conduct is grossly unprofessional and the practitioner unwilling to heed warnings, this should be reported to the professional body, which can take measures to deal with the matter. If the matter proceeds further and a practitioner is called upon by law or the professional body to provide evidence against another practitioner's professional conduct, only evidence that is pertinent to the case is required. Openly criticizing or slurring another practitioner is unacceptable and unethical, and jeopardizes the public's perception of the profession.

> *"10. No practitioner should advise, prescribe or engage in any procedure beyond his competence and training. Engaging in occasional practice is not in the best interests of the patient: practitioners should be aware of their limitations and refer to a more competent colleague as necessary."*

Optometrists should practise as optometrists. Some practitioners have acquired extra skills and specialize in various aspects of optometric practice. In order to retain specialist status, the practitioner needs to engage in this aspect of practice on a regular basis, to update knowledge and skills, and to keep abreast of advances in that particular area. Working once a month as a locum in a practice in which all other practitioners specialize in binocular vision does not entitle the locum optometrist to present him or herself as a binocular vision specialist. Acquisition of such skills cannot be by association. No shame should be attached to a practitioner who is not familiar with an area of practice that has become specialized. For example, not every optometrist prescribes or advocates orthokeratology. Practitioners who do not work in this area cannot be expected to know as much about it as those who do. If a patient comes in asking for more information about orthokeratology, they can be referred to a practitioner who specializes in prescribing this form of treatment.

The code of ethics for optometrists is not a set of rules but a series of guidelines to promote good practice. Its purpose is to make optometrists aware of their responsibilities towards patients, colleagues and other professionals, and to help each practitioner develop a set of personal ethics to which he or she adheres. As practitioners develop their own ethical practice and extend what is provided by the College of Optometrists, they may wish to contribute to developing the guidelines in order to advance ethics in optometric practice.

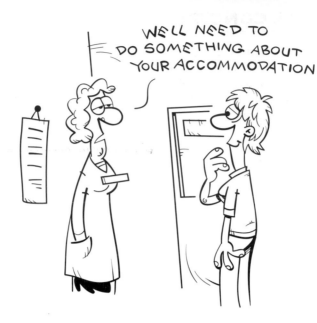

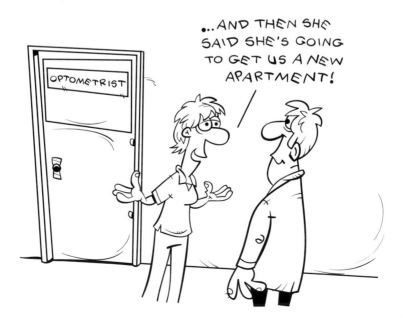

ETHICAL CONCEPTS

Ethical issues can be complex, and sometimes it is helpful to a separate an ethical matter into its basic components or concepts. This can aid in solving a problem or in making a clearer judgement about a particular situation. Ethical concepts that are relevant to healthcare practice are:

- virtues
- values
- rights
- respect
- dignity
- principles
- standards
- duties
- responsibility
- accountability

Virtues

These are admirable traits of character. In terms of professional practice, virtues are:

1. Competence in your expertise as an optometrist
2. Loyalty and trustworthiness towards patients and colleagues
3. Honesty in your dealings.

Values

Value is a matter of a state of affairs being good or bad, or being better or worse than another state of affairs. Improving the vision of a patient translates to replacing one state of affairs with a better state of affairs. A comparison of good and bad requires evaluation or a judgement of value.

In professional practice, the practitioner needs continually to evaluate what is good and what can be better. The aim should always be to improve situations that can be made better and to maintain situations that are good. For example, a patient comes in for routine examination. There is no change in prescription. This is evaluated as a good situation and it should be kept that way. If the patient had needed a change in prescription, the situation would be evaluated as one that could be improved and steps would be taken to remedy it. There may be more than one way to do this. Refractive error can be corrected with spectacles, contact lenses or, if the patient wishes it and risks are considered to be minimal, a permanent solution such as laser refractive surgery may be appropriate.

Rights

Rights are entitlements that a person can expect from another person, from an institution or from the state. These are called *claim rights* (Rainbolt 2006). A claim right is one in which a person can expect others, those who have a duty with regard to this claim right, to respect or to honour. Rights can also be freedoms to enjoy certain privileges or to engage in specific activities (Rainbolt 2006). These are *liberty rights*. There is no duty involved in a liberty right. The distinction between the two is illustrated by a simple example.

A person wishes to purchase a new house and requires some assistance with meeting the full cost. He approaches a bank to discuss a mortgage and after some negotiation a sum and means and method of payment are agreed. The loan is received and the house purchased. The bank expects the person who borrowed the money to honour the mortgage agreement. In this situation the bank has a *claim right* to the repayments and the borrower has a duty to make these as agreed. The borrower's right with regard to his house is a *liberty right*: he can refurbish and decorate it as he wishes and enjoy it as he pleases. He has no duty to anyone with this liberty right, and nobody owes him any duty.

With regard to healthcare practice, people in the United Kingdom have a claim right to treatment. Those who work pay taxes, and a proportion of these monies is put into health care by the government. The duty of the government is to supply this health care to the public. Any adult patient who is sufficiently competent to understand the nature and consequences of a certain treatment has an additional *liberty right* to accept or refuse a particular form of treatment.

Respect

Consideration given to another person, high regard or esteem in which a person holds another person are measures of respect. They are based on inherent characteristics of the person who is respected. Respect from others needs to be earned. In the context of the clinical situation, a practitioner needs to gain respect as a professional and as a practitioner from both colleagues and patients. Respect should also be returned to patients and colleagues: respect for their needs, their individuality, their opinions and the decisions that they make.

Dignity

Dignity is linked to respect and self-worth. It is a characteristic worthy of respect or honour. The dignity of another person is preserved when the person is accepted and respected. Patients who come to an optometrist are coming for help, advice and care. They can be in a vulnerable position with respect to dignity. Take the example of a distinguished elderly gentleman who comes to his optometrist with some distance vision problems. He perceives his complaint to be easily remedied with a stronger pair of spectacles. Instead he is diagnosed with senile macular degeneration. The news is too overwhelming. He breaks down in the consulting room and starts to cry. For this man, such a display of emotion may feel humiliating and undignified. He needs to be assured that this is a common reaction and that basic human emotions are not perceived as a slight on his dignity.

Principles

Ethics are sometimes described by using principles. Principles are generalizations that do not name or specify any individual or group and do not apply to any particular time or place. Examples of principles are the following:

- You should strive to help those in need.
- The welfare of children should take precedence over other considerations.
- One should protect the vulnerable.
- People should be respected.

Each of these principles serves to guide general actions. Principles do not impose any obligations or rules. There is no 'must' in a principle; the operative word is 'should'. If a principle is followed, it is not followed selectively. In other words, if a person believes that those in need should be helped, they would apply this principle regardless of the person in need, the time or the place. If one strives to help people, this applies at any time and in any place, not just on the third Tuesday of the month, if in London.

Standards

A standard is an established measure that sets a criterion for action or behaviour. For example, in health care there is a standard of care that is expected of practitioners. The regulation that a prescription that is more than 2 years old needs to be checked is an example of such a standard. Standards established by professional bodies provide a basic level of performance and service to which professionals must adhere. Ethical standards can and should be set at a higher level. How high this level should be will vary with individual practitioners.

Duties

Duties are obligations that we can impose on ourselves or have imposed on us by the nature of our situation: personal or professional. A practitioner has a duty of care to his or her patients. A person is likely to have duties at home, which have been agreed by the person and those with whom he or she lives. There are also duties that we are bound to follow if set by the government or made in law. It is the duty of every parent to ensure that their children attend school. Words such as 'ought', 'should' and 'must' are often used when making expressions of duty. A duty that a person has chosen for him or herself, or one that has a moral basis, is more likely to be a duty that 'should' be followed, for example to attend Church service once a week. Duties imposed by law are requirements that 'must' be met, for examples to drive at or below the speed limit.

Responsibility

Responsibility is often used interchangeably with duty. Duties tend to be more specific than responsibilities and to be applied to well defined actions. A practice manager will have specified managerial duties to perform as well as the responsibility for ensuring that other employees perform their duties. If a receptionist comes in late, telephones her boyfriend and is rude to patients, she is not performing her duties to the required standard. It is the responsibility of the practice manager to ensure that the receptionist does her duty.

Accountability

Accountability means having to explain and justify actions or decisions if asked to do so. An optometrist may find him or herself accountable to several different parties at once, to his or her patients, to other optometrists in the practice, to his or her employer. For example, records show that a patient came in to see the optometrist twice in the last week but it is not clear why. The optometrist would be expected to explain and to account for the two consultations. It does not mean that the optometrist has done anything wrong, just that they need to be able to justify their actions. Sometimes this justification is one that the decision-maker needs to make to him or herself, but this is no less important than a decision or action for which he or she needs to be accountable to another person. An ethical decision, particularly a difficult one, should be made only after careful consideration and thorough judgement of alternatives.

SUMMARY

Optometry is an established healthcare profession that has a code of ethics set by the professional body. The code is supported by ten principles that provide guidance for practitioners. Basic ethical concepts that apply to health care may also help in understanding practice-based ethics and in making decisions.

References

Bailey R N, Heitman E 2000 Ethics in clinical optometry. In: Bailey R N, Heitman E (eds) An optometrist's guide to clinical ethics. American Optometric Association, St Louis, pp 5–6

BBC News 2003a 'Shocked' judge swore at police BBC News 24 September 2003. Online. Available: http://news.bbc.co.uk/1/hi/england/north_yorkshire/3135996.stm

BBC News 2003b Drunk judge fined £800. BBC News 29 September 2003. Online. Available: http://news.bbc.co.uk/1/hi/england/north_yorkshire/3149386.stm

BBC News 24 2004 Hooligans jailed over fight plot. BBC News 24 7 May 2004. Online. Available: http://news.bbc.co.uk/1/hi/uk/3693885.stm

BBC News 2006 BNP teacher 'should be banned'. BBC News 14 July 2006. Online. Available: http://news.bbc.co.uk/1/hi/education/5179408.stm

College of Optometrists 2007 Code of ethics and guidelines for professional conduct 2007. Online. Available: http://www.college-optometrists.org/index.aspx/pcms/site.publication.Ethics_Guidelines.recent/

Jones S 2004 Former judge admits child porn charges. Guardian Unlimited 17 June 2004. Online. Available: http://www.guardian.co.uk/child/story/0,7369,1240407,00.html

Optometrists Association Australia 2007 Code of ethics. Online. Available: http://www.optometrists.asn.au/association/ethics

Rainbolt G 2006 Rights theory. Philosophy Compass 1(ET 003):1–11. Online. Available: http://www.blackwellpublishing.com/pdf/compass/PHCO_003.pdf

The Opticians Act 1989 (Amendment) Order 2005 Statutory Instrument 2005, No. 848. HMSO, London. Online. Available: http://www.opsi.gov.uk/si/si2005/20050848.htm

4

Beneficence/ non-maleficence

BENEFICENCE

This ethical principle, which dates back to the Hippocratic Oath, is about the performance of good deeds for others. In a clinical construct it translates to practitioners doing the best for their patients. Outside the clinic, practitioners ought to do their best to help others who may be in need. This may appear to be so obvious that it hardly needs stating. No healthcare practitioner would consider practising without striving to do the best for his or her patients. The complicating factor with this ethical principle is not whether there are any reasons not to practise with beneficence but with the difficulty in defining its limits. The doing of good deeds has no limits. For example, a practitioner should always take sufficient time to examine each patient and to conduct a thorough examination. However, just how good and how thorough that examination should be cannot be defined easily and will vary from practitioner to practitioner. It is therefore not possible to tell a practitioner exactly how beneficent he or she should be.

Just as it is difficult to put a limit on the maximum level of beneficence that can be expected of a practitioner, it is also difficult to define the opposite of good in order to avoid doing what may not be good. If asked to give an antonym to 'good', the common response would be 'bad'. In some cases it is easy to see what constitutes a good deed and what does not. This may apply when we say that it is always good to examine a patient thoroughly and that it is always bad to conduct an inadequate examination.

However, it is not universally true to say that because it is always good to do a certain act, then it is always bad not to do this act. For example, few people would dispute that it is good to donate to charity. If donating to charity is a good deed, does it therefore always follow that not donating to charity is bad? The answer is no. There may be good reasons why someone may not to wish to donate to a particular charity. He or she may not agree that it is a worthy cause or, quite simply, may not have any money to donate. In the realm of health care and medicine it is a good and noble act to donate an organ for transplantation. Should all eye care professionals, optometrists and ophthalmologists, therefore, set a good example and donate their corneas for transplantation? This would be seen as an act of beneficence but it is not one that can be expected of all practitioners. There are people who may not wish to donate their body parts to medicine or to science. They may have personal moral or faith-based reasons for this, and these reasons should be respected. Beneficence does not require a practitioner to do deeds with which he or she may feel uncomfortable.

Beneficence may also be limited by the wishes and/or behaviour of the patient. The practitioner may be placed a situation in which they cannot do the utmost good for a patient because the patient will not co-operate. For example, obesity is risk factor for many serious and chronic illnesses: diabetes, heart disease, stroke, bone and joint ailments. Obesity is also avoidable as it is caused largely by over-eating and a sedentary lifestyle. Ultimately it depends on the person who is obese to do something to reduce their weight. If an obese patient is given advice and offered help with weight reduction but refuses to comply, the doctor cannot have the patient incarcerated so that their food intake can be controlled until such time as the weight is reduced to an acceptable and healthy level. Such drastic measures may indeed be the very best that the doctor could do for this patient but this would require acts that are unacceptable in our society. It is not illegal to be obese and therefore a doctor has no right to deprive an obese patient of their liberty to over-eat.

A similar situation arises with smoking. There is no dispute that smoking is bad for health. It leads to serious conditions such as cancer and it exacerbates other illness such as diabetes. Take the example of a diabetic patient who is overweight and a heavy smoker. He presents to his optometrist complaining of poor vision. There are signs of diabetic retinopathy on the fundus. As part of the treatment and advice, the optometrist strongly recommends that the patient stops smoking. The patient says that this is not possible. He has tried over the years to do this but has always been unsuccessful and in any case it would lead to an increase in his weight that he cannot afford. To do the very best for such a patient would require the optometrist to take active steps to stop the patient from smoking. However, as with the doctor and the obese patient, there are limits on what the optometrist can do.

There are also limits to beneficence that each practitioner needs to decide for him or herself. Examinations and services provided to patients depend on a number of things: time allotted for appointments, the number of other staff available, the type of patients seen and their needs. One practitioner may decide that 30 minutes is ample time to conduct a thorough examination and to provide the best care that a patient needs. If there are further tests that need to be conducted then this practitioner will ask the patient to return on another day. Another practitioner may deem this to be insufficient time to do the very best for certain patients and may make appointments that are 45 minutes long to ensure that all necessary tests can be conducted on the same day. This would probably be more convenient for the patient, and the second practitioner may appear to be showing a greater level of beneficence. However, other factors need to be taken into account. Perhaps the first practitioner is working in a busy practice that is not her own and the appointment times have been fixed by the owner of the practice. She may not, therefore, be at liberty to make any changes and needs to do her best within the allotted time. The level of beneficence shown by these two practitioners cannot be compared.

The various forms of beneficence

To describe all acts of beneficence as being of a similar type (i.e. merely doing good) makes it difficult to define personal limits. Clearly there is a difference between conducting a thorough examination to meet patient needs and going beyond this to an entirely selfless practice that always puts the patients before family, personal life and any personal aspirations and ambitions that the practitioner may have. Beauchamp & Childress (2001) make the distinction between what they call obligatory and ideal beneficence. *Ideal beneficence* is the selfless form that includes sacrifice and the performance of such good and charitable deeds that would benefit all persons who come in contact with the practitioner. Mother Teresa was an example of an ideally beneficent individual who devoted her life to care for the poor and needy. Extreme levels of selflessness are not expected of healthcare practitioners. A form of beneficence that brings about good for patients but that does not require the practitioner to make extreme sacrifices in his or her personal life may be more appropriate and more sustainable. An ethical practitioner should aim to practise in a way that benefits his or her patients, but this can be balanced with a lifestyle that satisfies the practitioner's other needs and allows the fulfilment of duties outside the practice. This is not ideal beneficence but akin to the beneficence that Beauchamp & Childress (2001) call obligatory beneficence.

Case study

You are a happily married parent with two adult children who have left home and a 6-year-old boy. This youngest child has contracted a serious kidney infection and requires blood transfusions and a kidney transplant, or he will die. You have a matching blood type and would be the perfect donor. The operation and transfusion carry a 50% chance of success for your son. If he does survive, the chances of his body rejecting the transplant are 10% in the first 5 years, 30% in the following 10 years and up to 40% over 30 years. He will be on immunosuppressant drugs for the rest of his life. Your own survival, should you agree to the donation and transfusion, is estimated at less than 50%. The doctors are unable to provide you with an exact figure. Your spouse has left it to you to make the decision and will support whatever you decide to do.

- *Will you consent to the donation for any hope of saving your son's life?*
- *Would you decide otherwise if this was your eldest child and there were two younger siblings who required many more years of parental care?*
- *Would you decide otherwise if you were a single parent?*

The term *obligatory beneficence*, which has its basis in the philosophical writings of Jeremy Bentham and of William David Ross (Beauchamp & Childress 2001), may, however, be a little misleading. Beneficence, like any ethical principle, ought not to be considered purely as an obligation. This implies that it is practised because it is imposed by some external body or person, that it is a duty that must be fulfilled. Ethics cannot be practised merely as a duty. Although there is no dispute that there is a responsibility attached to providing a good-quality eye service, practising with beneficence should also include a level of care that is not imposed by any external factors but is decided by the practitioner. It should form an integral part of any practitioner's approach to patients and should be developed by each practitioner according to personal values and beliefs.

The virtue of compassion

Compassion is highlighted by Beauchamp & Childress (2001) as an expression of beneficence. To do the best for others requires not only concern for their welfare but also an understanding and sympathy for their situation and, wherever it occurs, for their suffering. Compassion, like beneficence, needs to be applied properly and cannot be unrestricted. The overly compassionate practitioner may misjudge a certain situation, resulting in an act that is not the best course of action for the patient. Beauchamp & Childress (2001) cite the case of a son who had been estranged from his father. The father was almost comatose and being kept alive by a very painful treatment that was of limited use. The son wanted this treatment to continue for however long it was necessary to allow him to make up with his father. Another relative wanted the treatment to end. Some of the staff at the hospital felt deep compassion for the son and thought that keeping the father alive was the right thing to do so that father and son could make their peace. Other staff felt that such compassion was ill-judged and that continuing to keep the father alive was wrong. He was suffering needlessly, his prognosis was very poor, and the equipment was needed to help other patients.

Compassion may need to be assessed at times to see that it is applied to the person who needs it without causing harm to others. Take the following case:

Clinical case study

A patient comes to see his practitioner for a routine eye examination. He is 58 years old and employed as a lorry driver travelling long distance to deliver items and products to warehouses and supermarkets. His best corrected visual acuity is 6/12 in one eye and 6/18 in the other. The fundus shows signs of diabetic retinopathy and the lenses in both eyes have nuclear yellowing and secondary cataracts. The patient is told that he cannot drive as his eyesight does not meet the requirements for driving. It is possible that vision will improve after the cataracts have been removed, but a second opinion about whether the lenses can be replaced in the near future is needed because of the fragile nature of the retina.

The patient becomes very distressed. He cannot afford to stop working. The company has made some of his friends redundant and any admission of ill-health or time taken to have an operation would leave him vulnerable and likely to lose his job. He claims that he knows the routes and, even though some journeys are long and require driving at night, he is confident that he will have no problems. He tells the practitioner he cannot and will not take any time off work and asks the practitioner not to report him to the driving standards authority.

To show compassion towards this patient does not mean complying with his wishes. Beneficence is about doing good deeds for the patient but not at the expense of safety. By allowing him to continue driving with deficient eyesight, the practitioner would be putting him in a situation that could lead to harm and injury to the patient and potentially to others. Beneficence in this case means acting against the patient's wishes: telling him that he should cease driving until vision can be improved. If, after a cataract extraction and implant replacement, vision is still under the required limit, he will have to stop driving and return his licence to the appropriate driving standard authority.

What the patient wants

Sometimes the actions that a doctor or healthcare practitioner takes may be focused entirely on doing what the patient wants, and this is considered to be in the best interests of the patient. However, satisfying the wishes of a patient may at times appear to disregard other people who may be directly or indirectly affected. The case of Dr Antinori and his patient Dr Patricia Rashbrook illustrates this situation.

Britain's oldest mother

In 2006, Dr Severino Antinori helped Dr Patricia Rashbrook to become pregnant at the age of 62 years, using in-vitro fertilization (IVF) treatment. On the 5 July 2006, Dr Rashbrook became Britain's oldest mother. Dr Antinori had made medical history and achieved acclaim for his skills. Dr Rashbrook already had adult children from a previous marriage. She wanted to have a baby to 'cement her marriage' to her second husband, who had no other children. As Dr Rashbrook was beyond the age of fertility, a donor egg had to be used. Dr Rashbrook was a child psychiatrist who could be expected to have a deep understanding of what is needed to maintain emotional and mental as well as physical well-being of a child. She was also a woman who could afford to pay for the expensive IVF treatment and to travel to Rome and Eastern Europe, with associated costs of care, to see Dr Antinori and to receive the treatment. Dr Rashbrook has been heavily criticized by many people, including members of her own family. She asked that her decision be respected as a private matter (BBC News 2006a).

This case has raised a number of fundamental questions and aroused much debate about the ethical and moral implications of offering IVF treatment to women who have passed the age at which they can conceive children naturally. Technological advances are sometimes made at such a rate that there is insufficient time to allow proper consideration of the underlying legal and ethical issues.

The questions arising from this case concern beneficence and patient wishes, but also delve further into the questions of whether medical science should interfere with nature:

- *Was Dr Antinori adhering to the principle of beneficence and doing his very best for one of his patients, or is it possible that Dr Antinori may also have had other motives? If so, can he still be considered to be acting in the best interests of his patient?*
- *Is it moral and ethical to traverse outside the boundaries of nature and try to have a child at an age when a woman is post-menopausal?*
- *Should the patient's wishes come first or should a talented doctor such as Dr Antinori concentrate his research efforts and skills on helping younger women with infertility problems? Dr Rashbrook already had children.*
- *Does this create inequalities in society because not everyone can afford to have the treatment at Dr Antinori's clinic, or should we consider the fact that an affluent couple like Dr Rashbrook and her husband will be able to provide the very best for their child?*

Continued

- *Is Dr Rashbrook being selfless by trying to cement her marriage or selfish because she has not considered the implications for the child? She will be in her eighties when her child finishes secondary education.*
- *Is wanting to strengthen a relationship a good enough reason for having a child? Biologically, the child is not Dr Rashbrook's as it was conceived with a donor egg.*
- *Just because a scientific or medical advance has been made, should it be available to all, even if that means going against what is natural?*
- *Should society be concerned about this at all, or should Dr Rashbrook's decision be respected as a private matter?*

Can beneficence include refusing treatment to patients?

It would seem to be the very antithesis of beneficence to refuse to offer treatment or care to a patient. However, there are instances where this may be the only and best method of helping the patient. Should a dentist continue to treat a child for tooth decay when the child refuses to stop eating sweets? Repeated treatment will not stop the cause but merely treat the effects. Given that a diet high in sugar has other detrimental consequences to the health of the child, refusal to treat until the diet is corrected may be the more beneficent act. A similar approach is being taken with regard to in-vitro fertilization (IVF) treatment and the recommendation by the British Fertility Society that this treatment should not offered to obese women (BBC News 2006b). These women have more problems with conception and IVF than women of healthy weight, and for the obese this treatment is less likely to be successful. In addition, the health risks associated with obesity are exacerbated by pregnancy. Offering this treatment to women who are already at risk of diabetes and high blood pressure may be harmful to them, and is therefore unlikely to be considered as an act of beneficence.

Similar situations can arise in eye care practice. A patient may wish to have contact lenses and may insist that this is the only prescription that is appropriate for his or her needs. The patient's standards of hygiene leave much to be desired and, in addition, previous contact lens wear has resulted in him or her presenting with giant papillary conjunctivitis. It is clear that contact lenses are contraindicated in such a case. To prescribe them to this patient on the basis that the patient believes that this serves his or her best interests is not beneficent. It is harmful.

NON-MALEFICENCE

Part of the Hippocractic Oath states: 'Above all to do no harm'. This defines non-maleficence: not to act in a way that will bring about bad consequences. Non-maleficence is related to beneficence in that both principles support the doing of good deeds. The major difference between non-maleficence and the principle of beneficence is that, because non-maleficence describes what should not be done, it does have limits. Avoiding harm, unlike doing good, is not limitless.

Like beneficence, non-maleficence may appear at first glance to be obvious. No healthcare practitioner would consider, wittingly, harming a patient. There are many instances, however, in which treatment or examination methods pose a risk for the patient. Non-maleficence requires that the good to be gained by these treatments or methods is not outweighed by any potential harm that may be caused. In medical practice, the prescription of medication and the use of surgery are examples where non-maleficence must be considered. Medication is rarely without side-effects and every surgical procedure carries risks. The question that must be addressed when prescribing and treating is: 'Do the benefits outweigh the risks?'. If the answer is 'yes' then the treatment is offered. Non-maleficence is about considering the risks of any treatment or method of care and comparing these to the benefits that the treatment may have for the patient.

Analysis of risks and benefits

The consideration of risks is inherent in most aspects of clinical practice. It starts with the case history. A patient is asked about their past medical history and about any medical conditions within their family. This informs the practitioner about the possibility of potential conditions that may arise and alerts him or her to prevailing conditions. For example, a 30-year-old patient presents for an eye examination and reveals, during the taking of the case history, that there is a family history of glaucoma. Although there may be no symptoms of the condition reported by this patient and she is below the age at which measurements of intraocular pressure are routinely conducted, this patient should have her intraocular pressures measured.

During the course of examination, practitioners look for signs that may contraindicate certain types of treatment. An elderly patient presents with a cataract that has caused a reduction in visual acuity in the right eye by one line on the Snellen chart since the patient was last seen 2 years ago. The patient has also had a retinal detachment in that eye and the corrected visual acuity for that eye has been $^6/_{18}$ since the operation to reattach the retina, 10 years ago. The patient relies on vision in the other eye, which has a corrected visual acuity of $^6/_{7.5}$. This has not altered since the last visit. Such a patient is unlikely to be referred for a cataract extraction. The benefit of a single line on the Snellen chart in the eye on which the patient does not rely is not worth the risk of operating on an eye that has had a detached retina.

Often there is more than one way of treating a condition. The choice of treatment will depend on what is the most suitable for the patient, but there may be situations where more than one type of treatment appears to be equally suitable and equally beneficial. Here the consideration of risk becomes paramount. The correction of myopia is an excellent example. Myopia can be corrected with spectacles, contact lenses and orthokeratology, or potentially eliminated by refractive surgery. The first three options are within the realm of the primary care practitioner. Spectacles pose the least risk but do not eliminate the error and are considered, by some, to be least aesthetically pleasing. Contact lenses may have a slightly higher risk in some patients but appeal to many because they are more convenient for sporting activities and the evidence of the correction is removed. Both spectacles and contact lenses are prescribed routinely and pose lower risks but require the wearing of a corrective aid. Orthokeratology offers the patient clear vision without having to wear a correction for a significant number of hours during the day. This is achieved by wearing a tight contact lens during the night when oxygen levels to the cornea are at their lowest. There is a risk (albeit low) of serious damage to the cornea, such as ulceration (Chen et al 2001, Hutchinson & Apel 2002) and the risks are greater for children (Young et al 2004). Such damage is not common and it has been suggested that orthokeratology may retard the progression of myopia if prescribed in the early school years (Cho et al 2005).

The benefits and the risks would appear to be greater for orthokeratology than for spectacle and contact lens wear. Benefit in this case needs to be defined clearly. What benefit is the patient seeking: to correct myopia, or to correct myopia without having to wear the correction during the day? Is that extra aspect, of being correction-free during the day, worth the greater risk that orthokeratology involves? The answers to these questions depend on the attitude and approach of the practitioner to risk assessment as well as on the suitability and the wishes of the patient. (It is not strictly correct to say that it also depends on the needs of the patient, because the patient's basic need is to correct the myopia. This can be done equally well with spectacles or contact lenses.) For some practitioners the risks would be considered too high and the benefits not sufficiently justified. For others, orthokeratology has shown good results and their patients are happy. The risks are considered to be minimal compared with the added benefit of corrected vision without the need for spectacles or contact lenses during the day.

The prevention of harm – the role of the patient

In a number of cases practitioners have to deal with situations and conditions that are induced or exacerbated by the patient. In some instances, a patient may be unaware that what they are doing has

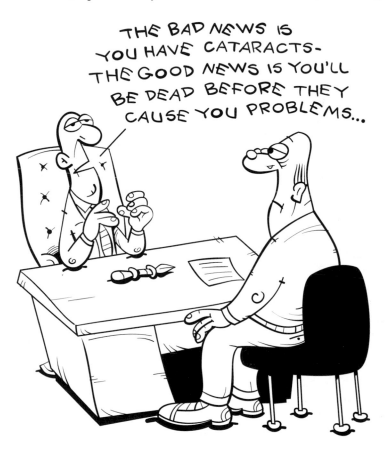

the potential for injury. Informing the patient of the dangers involved in their actions may be all that is needed. A simple example is of a patient who rubs their eyes excessively and presents with conjunctivitis. On examination, the patient is found to have superficial corneal staining. The patient needs to be told that rubbing of the eyes can lead to corneal damage and informed of the consequences of such damage. In other cases, the prevention of harm may be more difficult and the risk of harm less easy to predict.

Clinical case study

A young athletic patient presents to your clinic for a routine examination. During the course of the examination he mentions that he is travelling to New Zealand where he will be taking part in a bungee jumping competition. He had a traumatic sports injury to one eye a couple of years ago. This resulted in a retinal detachment that was treated successfully. You have heard that the jolt at the end of a bungee jump can be so abrupt that it can result in a retinal detachment. These appear to be rare occurrences, but you mention it to the patient. He asks you about the chances of this happening to him. This is a question that you are unable to answer. You have no information about the incidence of retinal detachment caused by bungee jumping and you do not know enough about the risk factors that may predispose a person to this happening. The best you can offer is the advice that bungee jumping has been reported as causing retinal detachments and that, given the fact that the patient has had a retinal detachment in the past, he may wish to be careful.

In some instances the potential harm can be identified, the patient advised either to take required steps or to desist from certain activities that increase the risk of harm, but the patient ignores the advice and warnings. In such situations, it is important to remember that total responsibility for preventing harm cannot always lie with the practitioner. With respect to illness, Hippocrates wrote:

> "The art consists in three things – the disease, the patient, and the physician. The physician is the servant of the art, and the patient must combat the disease along with the physician."
>
> (Hippocrates 400 BC)

The extent of responsibility accepted by the practitioner will vary with the practitioner, the patient, and the situation or condition.

Clinical case study

Bill is 30 years old and has keratoconus. The condition does not appear to be progressing and the current prescription has been stable for some years. He can attain a good level of visual acuity with spectacles and with gas-permeable contact lenses. He prefers the latter method of treatment. It is possible that the contact lenses are contributing to the non-progression of the condition but this is not certain. In spite of numerous attempts to explain the importance of hygiene and proper maintenance of contact lenses, Bill continues to neglect this aspect of care. He often wears the lenses for longer than the prescribed time and boasts that he has even fallen asleep without removing the lenses. Consequently he presents every few months with red, sore and itchy eyes that he rubs with abandon, even though he has been warned not to do this. Bill now requires a new pair of lenses, as he has lost one and the other is scratched. You wonder whether prescribing and providing Bill with a new pair of contact lenses is the right thing to do.

Should Bill be:

- warned, yet again, of the consequences of poor hygiene but provided with a new pair of contact lenses anyway? After all, he has been fully informed about the aspect of care over which he has control and its importance. If he ignores this, it is his choice.
- told that you will not provide him with another pair of contact lenses because the risk of damage to his cornea and potential acceleration of his condition is too great? He is, of course, at liberty to take his prescription to another practitioner who, unaware of Bill's attitude, is likely to prescribe contact lenses.
- told that it is better for his ocular health that he be prescribed a spectacle correction without specifying the exact reason, knowing that if Bill's attitude to contact lens hygiene is raised he will dismiss it?

The risk/benefit that has to be considered in this case is the risk of injury or damage that Bill is likely to cause himself against the possibility that the contact lenses are contributing to a slowing in progression of the keratoconus. The risk is evident, the benefit less clear. The keratoconus may have stopped progressing by itself, without the aid of the contact lenses. The prescription shows that the condition is not advanced and Bill is at an age when changes are not expected. However, if there is a benefit, it will be provided by the actions of the practitioner. The risk is derived from the actions, or inactions, of the patient. Whichever course of action is chosen, it needs to be justified.

The first option, which is to continue with the contact lenses, supports the benefit that may be provided. The potential benefits are considered to outweigh the risks, which, because they are avoidable, may in time be reduced. It is, after all, in the patient's interest to preserve his ocular health. This option takes a longer-term view and factors in the possibility that the patient may change his attitude.

The second option considers the risks as sufficiently serious and does not rely on the patient changing his approach to hygiene and care. The situation is taken as it is. The patient has not been adhering to the cleaning and care routines that are necessary. The practitioner is not going to continue with a treatment that is not being administered properly. This option not only highlights the risks, it puts the emphasis on the choice and responsibility of the patient. The contact lenses will not be prescribed because of the irresponsible attitude of the patient. The patient now has the choice of going to another practitioner.

The third option, like the second one, treats the risks as greater than any potential benefits. This time, the responsibility and all decision-making is left entirely up to the practitioner. The patient is not trusted to co-operate with the care regime and is therefore excluded from deciding the choice of treatment. If benefits are minimal or non-existent, this may be the safest option of all three, but it places the patient in a subordinate, almost child-like, position. It could be argued that, given the past actions of the patient, this is best way of eliminating risks. This choice of action is one in which the practitioner actively tries to prevent the patient from causing himself harm.

There is no right or wrong option. Each has its merits and weaknesses. It is for the practitioner to decide and to justify which they think is the best course of action.

Is prevention of harm an act of beneficence or non-maleficence?

The distinction between doing good and avoiding harmful acts was made in the writings of Hippocrates. What are now referred to as beneficence and non-maleficence are clearly distinguished in the reference to 'two special objects':

"The physician must be able to ... have two special objects in view with regard to disease, namely, to do good or to do no harm."

(Hippocrates 400 BC)

In many subsequent writings the two are recognized as separate ethical principles (Beauchamp & Childress 2001), whereas in others they are treated as one (Frankena 1973). There is also an uncertainty about whether preventing harm or protecting another person from harm should be considered under beneficence or non-maleficence. Beauchamp & Childress (2001) place the prevention or removal of harm under the principle of beneficence. This is because they interpret prevention or removal of harm as 'doing something' and that 'something' is a helpful act and hence an act of good. Non-maleficence, according to Beauchamp & Childress (2001), is the principle of 'not doing' something or desisting from an action. It could equally be argued that beneficence describes actively doing only good whereas non-maleficence is about acting to avoid doing harm. According to this line of argument, because preventing or removing harm has limits, it cannot be called beneficence as beneficence has no restriction.

Although this makes for an interesting and profound philosophical debate, it does not matter for practical purposes. When a practitioner refuses to prescribe contact lenses to a patient, for whom there are contraindications to contact lens wear, is he avoiding the risk of harm or is he actively protecting the patient from a potentially harmful choice? Either could be argued, and the consequence would be the same. Whether these are both acts of non-maleficence or whether one is an act of beneficence is unimportant. What is important is that the practitioner has behaved ethically.

SUMMARY

The principles of beneficence and non-maleficence are integral to clinical practice. They lead to duties to act in ways that will produce value or benefit. Beneficence, or doing the best for patients, is expected of every healthcare practitioner. Defining what is meant by 'the best', however, can be difficult. It can be complicated by patients' wishes and the unlimited nature of doing good. The limits have to be set by each practitioner and these limits will depend on personal values, lifestyle and the level of compassion that a practitioner possesses. Non-maleficence, or preventing harm and bad consequences, has more limits than beneficence. It requires a risk–benefit analysis and may involve the patient taking greater responsibility for his or her health. Whether the action of the practitioner is one of doing good, or one that aims to avoid or to prevent harm, the benefit should always be to the patient.

References

BBC News 2006a Briton becomes new mother at 62. BBC News 8 July 2006. Online. Available: http://news.bbc.co.uk/2/hi/health/5160142.stm

BBC News 2006b Call for fertility ban for obese. BBC News 30 August 2006. Online. Available: http://news.bbc.co.uk/1/hi/health/5296200.stm

Beauchamp T L, Childress J F 2001 Principles of biomedical ethics, 5th edn. Oxford University Press, New York

Chen K H, Kuang T M, Hsu WM 2001 Serratia Marcescens corneal ulcer as a complication of orthokeratology. American Journal of Ophthalmology 132(2):257–258

Cho P, Cheung S W, Edwards M 2005 The longitudinal orthokeratology research in children (LORIC) in Hong Kong: a pilot study on refractive changes and myopia control. Current Eye Research 30:71–80

Frankena W 1973 Ethics, 2nd edn. Prentice-Hall, Englewood Cliffs, NJ

Hippocrates 400 BC Of the epidemics (trans. F. Adams). Online. Available: http://classics.mit.edu/Hippocrates/epidemics.html

Hutchinson K M, Apel A 2002 Infectious keratitis in orthokeratology. Clinical and Experimental Ophthalmology 30:49–51

Young A L, Leung A T S, Cheng L L, Law R W K, Wong A K K, Lam D S C 2004 Orthokeratology lens-related corneal ulcers in children: a case series. Ophthalmology 111:590–595

5

Respect for autonomy

"... the only purpose for which power can be rightfully exercised over any member of a civilised community, against his will, is to prevent harm to others. His own good, either physical or moral, is not a sufficient warrant. He cannot rightfully be compelled to do or forbear because it will be better for him to do so, because it will make him happier, because, in the opinion of others to do so would be wise, or even right."

John Stuart Mill in *On Liberty*

A central principle in healthcare ethics, respect for autonomy, is respect for people and for their choices. An autonomous person is a person who has an understanding of their situation and is able to make their own plans and decisions, and to pursue personal goals. In short, autonomous people run their own lives. In the United Kingdom, mentally competent adults over the age of 18 years are considered by law to be autonomous individuals. There is an exception in healthcare practice, where the minimum age at which a patient can make his or her own decisions and give consent to treatment is 16 years (Family Law Reform Act 1969, section 8).

Although it is understood that autonomy means the right and/or the liberty to make a choice for oneself, in an organized society these choices need to be within the remit of laws and in accordance with regulations made by that society. We cannot do just as we please. If a person decides to walk out of a shop without paying for items that they have selected, they will be breaking the law and will be duly and appropriately punished. If a full-time employee decides not to come to work on Mondays because a weekend of 2 days is too short for their liking, the employee may do that without having committed any crime. However, they will in breach of a contractual obligation with the employer and there is likely to be a consequence that will result in the person becoming unemployed. Absolute freedom of choice cannot exist in an organized society. Choices must take into account the impact that they may have on others. Each of us, therefore, has a level of autonomy located somewhere on a continuum between perfect autonomy and no autonomy at all.

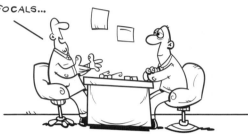

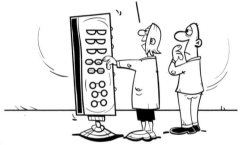

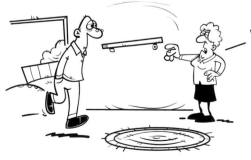

In healthcare practice, respect for autonomy means respecting patients, their choices and their opinions. It also means that these choices need to be informed. Patients should be provided with all the relevant information they need before they can make a choice. It is no good asking a patient whether they prefer multifocal lenses with a photochromic tint to two pairs of single vision spectacles with a polarizing clip-on for the distance vision pair, without explaining exactly what the difference is, the effect of each choice and the respective costs.

The principle of autonomy and the requirement to inform patients about their condition and treatment and to seek consent is relatively recent (Beauchamp 1997). It does not appear in the writings of Hippocrates and even as recently as the 19th century the famous treatise on medical ethics by Thomas Percival did not include autonomy (Beauchamp 1997). It is gaining greater recognition as patients are made more aware of their rights and this ethical principle has developed together with the law. Hence, the application of the respect for autonomy has some guidance in legislation and from decisions made in common law.

INFORMING PATIENTS ABOUT CONDITIONS AND TREATMENT OPTIONS

Informing a patient does not mean having to tell the patient absolutely everything there is to know about a condition. It means explaining the salient points and in such a way that the patient understands. This will vary depending on the patient, on their level of comprehension, on their familiarity with the English language and, in part, on their interest. Some patients may wish to know more about a certain condition and approach the interaction with the clinician as an opportunity to learn about any ailment or condition they may have. Other patients may wish to know only the basic information that will help them to make a choice. Having explained the nature of a condition or treatment, there should be no expectation on the patient to remember what they have been told. A clinical examination is not a teaching exercise. A patient may misunderstand or simply forget what has been said – and even that it was ever said. If it is important that a patient remembers, the practitioner should make a note that the patient has been informed. It may also be useful to ask the patient to sign this note.

INFORMING PATIENTS ABOUT RISKS

Some treatments are not without risk and patients need to be informed about these or any other side-effects and, if possible, about the chances of an adverse occurrence. Informing patients about risks has grounding in common law, notably from the case of Sidaway v Board of Governors of Bethlem Royal Hospital [1985].

Sidaway v Board of Governors of Bethlem Royal Hospital [1985]

Sidaway had undergone an operation on her cervical vertebrae, the outcome of which resulted in severe damage to her spinal cord. Sidaway claimed that she had not met with the surgeon before the operation and therefore had not been informed of the risks. The procedure was known to carry some risk, albeit small, and it was found that the surgeon had explained the risk of damage to the nerve root but had not discussed the risk of damage to the spinal cord. The Law Lords who heard the case recognized the need to inform patients about risks that are known or where the risks are 'real' or 'material':

"... a patient has a right to be informed of the risks inherent in the treatment which is proposed."
> (Lord Scarman, Sidaway v Board of Governors of Bethlem Royal Hospital [1985] – Howarth & O'Sullivan 2000)

but also recognized that the risks, particularly where they are not high, may at times be difficult for a patient to understand:

"A doctor cannot set out to educate the patient to his own standard of medical knowledge of all the relevant factors involved."
> (Lord Bridge of Harwich, Sidaway v Board of Governors of Bethlem Royal Hospital [1985] – Howarth & O'Sullivan 2000)

Lord Scarman also noted that, even if the risk was material but the doctor considered that informing the patient of the risk would be damaging to the health of the patient, the doctor would not be held liable for withholding this information. Similar guidance regarding disclosure of information about risks to patients has been issued by the General Medical Council (1998).

In eye care practice the same guidance should apply. A patient should be informed of risks but not unduly alarmed by the prospect of a risk that may be very small. The understanding that the patient has with regard to what he or she has been told is vital. Informing the patient of a risk that they do not comprehend could result in the patient refusing to undergo an examination that has minimal or even negligible risk, but that might be necessary for proper diagnosis. Take the case of a patient over the age of 40 years with a family history of glaucoma who presents at an optometric practice. His intraocular pressures should be measured. Contact tonometry is the only method available in the practice and the practitioner explains to the patient that a probe will be touching the surface of his eye. The practitioner goes on to say that sometimes this may cause a slight abrasion to the surface and in rare instances this may lead to an inflammation. Although all of this may be true, the practitioner's frankness frightens the patient who subsequently refuses to have a pressure measurement conducted. The patient's choice in such a case will have been one based on unnecessary alarm. The risk of an abrasion caused by tonometry should be very small and avoidance of the risk achievable, as it depends on the competency of the practitioner. Any risks in the measurement of intraocular pressure also need to be compared with the risks of not making that measurement and allowing a potential case of glaucoma to be left without diagnosis and subsequent treatment. These risks have to be assessed by the practitioner before deciding what to tell the patient.

Although some risks depend on the skills of the practitioner, other risks are not so easily controlled. The risks of a contact lens wearer developing an infection may be small, but they do exist. Whether or not an infection does develop depends on a number of factors that the practitioner cannot control (the approach of the patient to hygiene) or even predict (physiology of the cornea and biochemistry of the tears). These risks have to be balanced against the benefits of the treatment, and both risks and benefits should be explained to patients before they can make an informed decision.

CAN PATIENT CHOICES ALWAYS BE RESPECTED?

Sometimes it can be very difficult to respect the choices made by a patient. This occurs when the patient is continuing with actions that are detrimental to their health in spite of being informed and warned of the consequences. In such cases, respect for autonomy is not the reason that a patient is permitted to continue with a choice of lifestyle that has grave consequences for their health. It is rather because there is no law that allows the medical or health-care practitioner to intervene and prevent a patient from a course of action that can lead to illness or harm. If such laws existed, the principles of beneficence and non-maleficence would compel the practitioner to take steps to intervene. In fact, the law respects the right of a person to make a choice about their health even if this appears to be against reason.

"the patient's right of choice exists whether the reasons for making that choice are rational, irrational, unknown or even non-existent."
Lord Donaldson in the case of Re T (Adult: refusal of medical treatment) [1992]

The lifestyle choice of the heavy smoker who presents with diabetic retinopathy and makes comments that suggest he is not following the recommendations made by his doctor cannot be respected. His right to make a choice, however, must be acknowledged, and he should continue to be warned about the consequences of his choices, even if these warnings have been issued in the past and gone unheeded.

The frustration that a practitioner may feel by the poor choices made by a patient is magnified many times when the person who is ill is a close relative. Respect for autonomy of a loved one can be severely tested and become very difficult to maintain when that person has chosen a course of action that is harmful and could be fatal.

Case study

You are happily married with three children, two boys and a girl. The girl has always been a child who is ambitious and driven. She is also keen to please parents and authority figures, and is quite vulnerable and sensitive. The approach you and your spouse have taken in raising your children has involved teaching the children the importance of respect for others, their choices and their opinions. Any problems and differences have been resolved through discussion. Since the age of 13, your daughter has been concerned with her body shape and has started to diet excessively in the past year. She is now 16 years old and is pitifully thin. You and your spouse are extremely concerned. She yields to your pressure to eat and you find it unusual that her

Continued

weight continues to drop. One day her brother reports that he has heard her vomiting in the bathroom after meals. When he questioned her, she denied it. You and your spouse broach the subject with her and she becomes extremely distressed. Your GP is concerned about her and refers her to a psychiatrist. She refuses to go as she does not accept that there is anything wrong with her and she is not 'going mental'. She also threatens to kill herself if she is made to undergo psychiatric assessment and forced to eat. She says she would 'rather be dead than be fat'.

The GP suggests that there is one option which may save your daughter but warns you that it is drastic and not without consequences. There is a body of literature that suggests that anorexia can be considered to have a component of mental illness. Although at age 16 she is considered to be an adult for the purposes of medical treatment, if she is deemed to be mentally incompetent she can be treated against her will. If you are prepared to have your daughter certified as (temporarily) mentally incompetent she can be transferred to a hospital where she will be treated.

- *Would you resort to this measure or would you respect her autonomy and continue to try to convince your daughter to make a choice to seek help and treatment? As she is the sort of child who always wants to please her parents, perhaps she will eventually do as you wish. There is a risk that she may also become very worried that you are unhappy with her actions and this could lead to further distress and hiding her behaviour.*
- *Will you be prepared potentially to cause her mental harm and distress (and risk a suicide attempt) by having her certified and forcibly treated in order to prevent further physical harm which, if left untreated, will be fatal?*
- *Would your answer be different if the person suffering from anorexia was not your daughter but (a) a sister or (b) a distant relative?*

THE LIMITS OF RESPECT FOR AUTONOMY

Just as society imposes limits on the choices we make, it also restricts our right to do with our bodies as we please. In the United Kingdom, the right to life is legally recognized and protected (The Human Rights Act 1998, Schedule 1, Article 2). However, this right to life does not extend to helping a person end their life. Even in cases of extreme pain, where a person has months to live and would like to alleviate their suffering, the law forbids assisted suicide.

The case of Diane Pretty

Diane Pretty was afflicted with a degenerative disease of the muscles. There was no known cure and Diane's condition progressed until she was paralysed, unable to speak clearly and required feeding via a tube. She was not expected to live for long and did not want to live out the short time she had left in suffering and in a state that she considered to deprive her of her dignity. She was unable to end her life, and wanted her husband to assist her in doing this. The law in the United Kingdom does not forbid suicide but it does forbid assisted suicide (Suicide Act 1961). If Diane's husband had helped her to die he would have been prosecuted.

Diane challenged this legal situation under the Human Rights Act 1998, claiming that the law preventing her from being allowed to die was an infringement of her human rights. This argument was rejected by all of the courts in the UK, so Diane took her case to the European Court of Human Rights (Pretty v UK [2002]). Here again her case did not succeed. Diane died on 11 May 2002.

Cases such as Diane Pretty's and other terminally ill patients, who are forced to live in pain and who have asked for the right to end their lives, have prompted calls for voluntary euthanasia to be legalized in the United Kingdom. Lord Joffe introduced the Assisted Dying for the Terminally Ill Bill, which is an attempt to allow an end to life where there is 'unbearable suffering'. The definition of *unbearable suffering* is given as:

> "*suffering whether by reason of pain, distress or otherwise which the patient finds so severe as to be unacceptable*" (s13(1)).

The Bill was defeated in the House of Lords on 12 May 2006 and is to be reintroduced. It remains to be seen whether this Bill will ever be passed. This is an extremely controversial area and has aroused much heated debate because it touches on the very essence of being and what this means in our society. The sanctity of life, which is held to be so precious in the United Kingdom, has always been considered to be absolute: we do not stop valuing life and cease protecting it when living may have become unbearable. Yet how very different can this value for life appear to the terminally ill person who is in terrible pain, and to relatives who are watching a loved one suffer. People in these circumstances, just like Diane Pretty, may feel that their autonomy is not being respected.

REFUSAL OF TREATMENT

Although a person may not be actively assisted to die, any mentally competent adult has the right to refuse treatment even if such refusal could result in death. This was shown in the case of B.

The case of B

B was an educated and mentally competent woman who suffered a haemorrhage in her spine that, 2 years later, led to her becoming a tetraplegic. In order to stay alive, B needed to be treated with a ventilator. She asked that this be removed. Hospital psychiatrists were undecided about whether she was mentally capable of making such a decision: some thought she was, others disagreed. She brought her case to court, where it was ruled that her autonomy should be respected. This case highlighted the fact that there is no right to use artificial means of keeping a patient alive if the patient does not wish to be kept alive in this way. (Re B (Adult: refusal of treatment) [2002])

With regard to eye care practice, there are rarely situations that require life-saving decisions, but this does not mean that they will never arise.

Clinical case study

A patient presents to your practice for a routine investigation. Ophthalmoscopic examination shows a strange pigmentation on the fundus of the right eye that appears to indicate a tumour. You refer the patient and your initial diagnosis is confirmed. The patient returns to you in tears, saying that he has been advised the eye must be removed or the cancer will spread further. He refuses to undergo this treatment, saying he would rather be dead than without an eye.

Ultimately, the patient's decision must be respected, but would you respect this choice or would you try to convince the patient to change his mind?

In most instances in eye care practice, the most serious consequences of refusal to be treated may be sight-threatening. If an elderly patient with advanced cataracts and visual acuity of ⁶⁄₆₀ in one eye and ⁶⁄₃₀ in the other eye refuses to have an operation to remove her lenses, this decision has to be respected. However, her visual needs and the effect of her impairment on others must also be considered. If she still insists on driving, she must be warned that this is against the law. If she refuses to acknowledge this, the practitioner should inform her that she is obliged to report the matter to the appropriate authority in the interests of her safety as well as that of the public.

Any refusal by a patient of treatment that the practitioner recommends should be recorded. The reason why the patient has refused should be investigated and noted, and it is advisable to have such a record signed and dated by the patient. This safeguards the practitioner in case, at a later date, the patient denies refusing treatment or a third party questions why the condition was not treated.

CHILDREN AGED BELOW 16 YEARS AND THE CONCEPT OF GILLICK COMPETENCY

Children aged less than 16 years have no legislative right to make their own decisions regarding medical or healthcare treatment. In general, parents or other adults who have parental responsibility in law should make the decision for the child. There is, however, a provision that originates from common law and the famous case of Gillick v West Norfolk and Wisbech Area Health Authority [1985] which permits a young patient, below the age of 16 years, to make a decision about treatment. Mrs Victoria Gillick, the mother of five daughters, wrote to her local health authority (LHA) requesting an assurance that the LHA would not prescribe contraception to or perform an abortion on any of her daughters (at the time all aged below 16 years) without obtaining her consent. The LHA refused to give this assurance, prompting Mrs Gillick to commence proceedings against the authority. Mrs Gillick felt very strongly that parents have the right to be informed and duty to decide about birth control measures offered to their daughters who are under the age of 16, and that these rights should be respected. Mrs Gillick took her case as far as the House of Lords (the highest court in the United Kingdom at the time). Of the five Law Lords who presided over this case, a majority of three decided against Mrs Gillick. However, the actions of Mrs Gillick and the subsequent rulings of the Law Lords led to the establishment of what is now known as 'Gillick competency' (sometimes referred to as 'Fraser competency' after the guidelines set out by one of the Law Lords who heard the case).

Gillick competency is ascribed to a child, under the age of 16 years, who is considered to be sufficiently mature to understand the nature and consequences of a treatment of procedure and to give consent to its application. Gillick competency originated from a case dealing with the prescription of contraceptive methods to young girls, and this is still the area of health care in which it is most applied. It does, however, extend to other areas of medical and health-care practice.

The difficulty with Gillick competency is that the law has left it to the practitioner to decide whether or not a young patient is Gillick competent. If such a decision is made, the practitioner has to treat the child as an autonomous adult. Parental consent is not required and, only if the child permits it, can parents be informed about any aspects of the condition, care and treatment. There are no guidelines for deciding competency, but any practitioner who deems a young patient to be Gillick competent should be prepared to justify this, should it ever be required.

Young people vary enormously in their maturity and capacity to understand. It may be difficult not to consider treating, as Gillick competent, a 15-year-old who brings her 1-year-old child for an eye examination and who has been estranged from her parents. She may be below what legislation deems to be an adult, but she has the responsibility for a dependant. She has to make decisions for her child and it would therefore also be reasonable to respect the decisions she makes for herself.

In general, eye care practitioners may prefer to err on the side of caution and seek parental consent for treatment of all patients under the age of 16 years. In many cases, the spectacles, contact lenses or other ocular treatments prescribed for patients aged less than 16 years are paid for or subsidized by parents. To expect a parent to pay for a prescription without informing them of the reason or need for a prescription, and without seeking their consent, could be considered somewhat unreasonable.

The provision of a right for children under 16 years of age to consent to treatment does not extend to the right to refuse treatment. If a child aged less than 16 years refuses a treatment, and the consequences of that refusal may lead to the child dying or becoming permanently disabled, the decision of the parents, or ultimately the Court, can override that of the child, regardless of how mature that child is held to be. This has occurred in some cases in which children who were of the Jehovah's Witness faith refused life-saving blood transfusions. The Court ruled against the wishes of the children, deeming them to be incompetent to understand the consequences of refusal (Re E [1993], Re S [1994], Re L [1998]).

ADULTS WHO MAY BE UNABLE TO EXERCISE AUTONOMY

The respect for autonomy of adults who may not be competent to make their own decisions and give consent to treatment is ethically difficult and legally unclear. A very sobering case, which highlighted the ethical and legal difficulties in gaining consent on behalf of a mentally incompetent adult, was the case of F [1989].

F v West Berkshire Health Authority

F was a woman in her thirties who was mentally disabled. She had a verbal capacity of a 2-year-old child and the mental capacity of a 4-year-old. She had been a voluntary inpatient at her local hospital for about 20 years, and at this hospital had formed a sexual relationship with a male mentally handicapped patient. It appeared to staff that she had physical enjoyment from the act of intercourse with this patient and that this was consensual. Staff did not wish to deprive her of this pleasure but recognized that fact that F could become pregnant. She was, however, mentally unable to understand the concept of childbirth and could not be prepared for the pain associated with giving birth. F was unable to take any form of contraception. Her mother, together with the doctors, agreed that it would be best to have F sterilized.

A declaration was requested from the courts to do this, and the lower courts agreed that sterilization would be in F's best interest. However, the Official Solicitor, who was brought in to act on behalf of F, appealed the decision. The judges had to consider the principle of autonomy and the fact

Continued

76

that F was an adult. There was a further important issue: sterilization was not a procedure that was needed to benefit F's health or to treat an underlying condition. Physically, F was healthy and an operation to sterilize her would require operating on a healthy organ to prevent it from functioning. For any mentally competent female, sterilization is a treatment that the patient elects. F was unable to make such a choice. The judgment addressed not whether it was acceptable to operate without F's consent, but whether, because F was unable to give consent, she should be deprived of treatment. Permission to perform the operation was ultimately granted as it was considered to be in the best interests of the patient.

This case raised the question of how mentally ill a patient needs to be in order to be considered unable to make his or her own decisions. The case of C offered some guidance (Re C [1994]).

C suffered from paranoid schizophrenia and was held in a mental hospital. He developed gangrene in his left leg. The doctors who examined him were convinced that if the leg were not amputated C would die. C thought otherwise. He had a belief that he was a medical expert of international standing and in his opinion the leg did not need to be amputated. C therefore refused the treatment and the matter went to Court. The Court ruled in C's favour and provided the following guidelines for deciding competency to consent to or to refuse treatment. A patient can be considered to be competent to consent to or to refuse treatment as long as they are able to:

- understand and remember information about the treatment;
- believe what has been said; and
- consider the options and make a decision.

Fortunately for C, he made a full recovery (Butler-Schloss 2006).

Frail or elderly patients may not be mentally incompetent but may be incapable of hearing properly and therefore of understanding what has been said. They may be forgetful and/or fearful of making a decision. They may be uncertain of which option to choose. In such cases communication must be clear, and greater care and patience are needed to impart the information to the patient and help them make a choice. Sometimes an elderly patient may be accompanied by one of their children or a carer. The elderly patient may prefer to have their child or carer with them in the clinic because this makes them feel more secure. An elderly patient may have a better understanding of information when it is imparted by a loved one or by someone on whom they rely. The accompanying child or carer may also be able to retain details that the elderly patent may forget. It should not be assumed that the presence of a child or carer indicates that the elderly patient is unable to make their own decisions. A frail or elderly patient may be vulnerable but should not be presumed to be less autonomous than any other adult patient. Denying such a patient respect for autonomy serves to increase their vulnerability:

> *"To presume that the incompetent person must always be sub-jected to what many rational and intelligent persons may decline is to downgrade the status of the incompetent person by placing a lesser value on his intrinsic human worth and vitality."*
>
> (from the judgment of the Supreme Judicial Court of Massachusetts in the case of Superintendent of Belchertown State School v Saikiewicz [1977] – Howarth & O'Sullivan 2000, p 752)

In eye care practice, even autonomous adults can be vulnerable and this vulnerability can increase with the severity of the condition. A patient with a progressively degenerating condition is likely to be uncertain and even to feel frightened about the future and how they will cope. The prospect of sight loss and dependency on another can make a person feel extremely vulnerable. The uncertainty about rate of progression of the condition and the level of loss that may occur can make any decisions difficult. The practitioner needs to be sensitive to the needs of such a patient and to show empathy and awareness of the patient's ability or inability to make a decision. The autonomy of the patient must continue to be respected, together with the recognition that such a patient may need more help and guidance with decision-making.

> *"All patients should be treated with courtesy and sensitivity to their individual needs."*
>
> (College of Optometrists 2007)

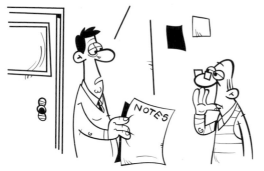

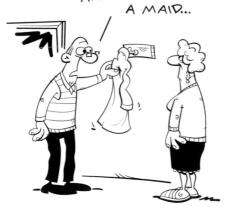

IN WHOSE BEST INTERESTS?

When decisions about health care or treatment are made for patients who are unable or not permitted to make their own decisions, the legal and ethical justifications are that the decision should be in the best interests of patient. Deciding what may be in the best interests of another person is never easy. It is particularly difficult when the other person is not capable of making any contribution to the decision and will never be capable of so doing. Young children grow up and could, as adults, challenge a decision made for them by their parents or guardians. A mentally incompetent person may never be able to do this, leaving such a person extremely vulnerable. When treatment is necessary for the health of such a person it may be justifiable. However, there are times when decisions are made to operate on a vulnerable person and yet the procedure offers no health benefits for this person. The 'best interests' argument is invoked but it is open to interpretation and debate. In whose best interests was the decision to operate on Y?

The case of Y

Y was physically and mentally disabled and was cared for in a nursing home. Her sister developed leukaemia and a bone marrow transplant was recommended to save her life. Y was the only member of the family whose marrow was compatible. There was a small risk to Y from the procedure and no health benefit for her. The court ruled that taking marrow from Y was in her best interests because, if Y's sister died, Y's mother would have to take care of the sister's child and would have less time to visit Y. (Re Y (Mental incapacity: bone marrow transplant) [1996])

Sometimes it is worth reflecting on how we, as a society, as individuals and as healthcare practitioners, view the vulnerable – those who are unable to speak, act and decide for themselves. When treatment is recommended for such patients, practitioners should always try to consider whether this is truly in the best interests of the patient and try to justify why this is so. This can be extremely difficult at times, and there may be no single best decision. The important point to remember is that this person deserves the respect given to any other patient, respect for their condition and respect for their dignity.

Clinical case study

A mentally disabled patient with severely impaired vision is brought to your clinic. The practitioner who usually visits her regularly is on maternity leave and the care home thought it would be in her best interests not to wait until the regular practitioner returned. There is no specific reason offered for the visit other than that a regular examination is due.

The patient appears to be extremely distressed and clearly does not want you to approach her. She seems particularly fearful of bright lights. The carer, who is not a relative, asks you to ignore this behaviour, telling you that the patient is often fretful in new situations.

Would you continue to examine this patient or would you recommend that the examination be postponed until the regular practitioner returns?

THE RIGHTS OF THE VULNERABLE

Members of society who are more vulnerable than others – children, the elderly, those who lack mental competence – require protection. The law offers some guidance about how to deal with issues of consent when treating such patients and this takes into account the best interests of the patient. There are instances in which vulnerable people are subjected to treatment or put in circumstances that are detrimental to their health, and society is limited in what it can do to protect these people. This happens when adverse treatments or circumstances are imposed by those on whom the vulnerable person depends. It occurs most commonly with children.

A parent, particularly of young children, who insists on smoking in their presence is exposing these children to the risk of harm. The detrimental effects of passive smoking are well documented. At present there is no law that protects these children. Legislation covers the prevention of smoking in public and workplaces but it does not extend to what is permitted or not permitted in the home. If it did, there would be cries of state intervention in personal life and accusations of an erosion of civil liberties. This would be an infringement on the principle of autonomy. It may also be challenged legally under Article 8 of the Human Rights Act 1998, which protects the Respect for Private and Family Life. Yet, by not restricting habits that pose a risk to health, vulnerable members of society are not being protected from these risks.

Article 8 of the Human Rights Act 1998

" 1. Everyone has the right to respect for his private and family life, his home and his correspondence.
2. There shall be no interference by a public authority with the exercise of this right except such as is in accordance with the law and is necessary in a democratic society in the interests of national security, public safety or the economic well-being of the country, for the prevention of disorder or crime, for the protection of health or morals, or for the protection of the rights and freedoms of others."

The second part of Article 8 leaves open the possibility for interference by a public authority if, among other exceptions, it is for the protection of health.

Smoking is not the only lifestyle habit that is dangerous; other habits may be even more difficult to control. Although smoking is an acknowledged risk to health for the smoker and others who are exposed to the smoke, and there is no need for anyone to smoke nor any benefit to be gained by engaging in the habit, eating is a somewhat different matter. Eating is necessary for survival and what a person eats, how much a person eats, when and where a person eats has no effect whatsoever on the health of another person. Yet, the type and amount of food consumed has a highly significant impact on health. Poor nutrition and overeating can lead to chronic illness. An autonomous person can decide what and how much he or she eats; a child is not capable of doing this. Childhood obesity in the United Kingdom, as in many countries in the developed world, is rising at an alarming rate (Ebbeling et al 2002). What a child eats and how much food a child consumes depends, to some extent, on the parents or guardians. To protect children fully from unhealthy eating habits would require the state dictating to parents what and how much they should feed their children. Again, and possibly even more vehemently than with smoking, the arguments about restrictions on civil liberties would be raised and a potential breach of Article 8 of the Human Rights Act 1998 could be invoked. It is worthy of note that when a school in South Yorkshire adopted healthy lunches for the children some mothers interpreted this as an act of infringement on the rights of those children to eat what they wanted. They posted themselves outside the school taking lunch orders and returning to supply children with fast foods and fizzy drinks (Stokes 2006).

As there is no government legislation that forbids exposing children or other vulnerable members of society to certain unhealthy habits, there is little that healthcare practitioners can do. Wherever possible and whenever appropriate, the practitioner should try to educate patients about the risks posed by unhealthy lifestyles and habits as well as about the consequences on the health of vulnerable people who may be affected.

SUMMARY

Respect for autonomy is a fundamental ethical principle in health care that has some guidance in law. In order for patients to exercise their autonomy they must be properly informed about the nature of the condition, the treatment options, the risk and benefits. How much information is given is up to the practitioner. Sometimes patients make informed decisions that are detrimental to their health. In such cases, the respect for the right of that patient to make the choice should not diminish, even though the practitioner may not agree with the choice. Children and vulnerable adults who are not able to make decisions about treatment must be protected as far as is possible. Any decisions made for them must always consider their best interests.

References

Assisted Dying for the Terminally Ill Bill (presented to the House of Lords, 9 November 2005. United Kingdom Parliament). Online. Available: http://www.publications.parliament.uk/pa/pabills/200506/assisted_dying_for_the_terminally_ill.htm

Beauchamp T L 1997 Informed consent in medical ethics. In: Veatch R M (ed.) Medical ethics: an introduction to medical ethics, 2nd edn. Jones & Bartlett, Sudbury, MA, p 185–209

Butler-Schloss E 2006 Legal aspects of medical ethics. Web Journal of Current Legal Issues 2 Web JCLI. Online. Available: http://webjcli.ncl.ac.uk/2006/issue2/butlersloss2a.html

College of Optometrists 2007 Code of ethics and guidelines for professional conduct (Professional Integrity 01.16). Online. Available: http://www.college-optometrists.org/index.aspx/pcms/site.publication.Ethics_Guidelines.recent/

Ebbeling C B, Pawlak D B, Ludwig D S 2002 Childhood obesity: public-heath crisis, common sense cure. Lancet 360:473–482

F v West Berkshire Health Authority and another (Mental Health Act Commission intervening) Re F (Mental Patient Sterilisation) [1989] 2 All ER 545

Family Law Reform Act 1969 The UK Statute Law Database, Ministry of Justice. Online. Available: http://www.statutelaw.gov.uk/Home.aspx

General Medical Council 1998 Seeking patients' consent: the ethical considerations (guidance document). Online. Available: http://www.gmc-uk.org/guidance/current/library/consent.asp#best_interests

Gillick v West Norfolk and Wisbech Area Health Authority [1985] UKHL 7, [1986] 1 FLR 229, [1986] AC 112. Online. Available: http://www.bailii.org/

Howarth D R, O'Sullivan J A 2000 Hepple, Howard and Matthews' tort: cases and materials, 5th edn. Butterworths, London, pp 328–333, p 752

Human Rights Act 1998 Office of Public Sector Information. Online. Available: http://www.opsi.gov.uk/acts/acts1998/19980042.htm

Mill J S 1859 On liberty. In: Warnock M (ed.) Utilitarianism, On Liberty and Essay on Bentham. Collins, Glasgow, 1979, pp 126–251

Pretty v UK [2002] 35 EHRR 1

Re B (Adult: refusal of treatment) [2002] 2 FCR1; [2002] 2 All ER 449 [2002] 1 FLR 1090, [2002] 2 FCR 1, 65 BMLR 149

Re C [1994] 1 WLR 290

Re E [1993] 1 FLR 386

Re L [1998] 2 FLR 810

Re S [1994] 2 FLR 1065

Re T (Adult: refusal of medical treatment) [1992] 4 All ER 649 at 662, (1993) Fam 95

Re Y (Mental incapacity: bone marrow transplant) [1996] BMLR 111 [1996] 2 FLR 329

Sidaway v Board of Governors of Bethlem Royal Hospital [1985] 1 All ER 643, [1985] AC 871, [1985] UKHL 1. Online. Available: http://www.bailii.org/

Suicide Act 1961 The UK Statute Law Database, Ministry of Justice. Online. Available: http://www.statutelaw.gov.uk/Home.aspx

Stokes P 2006 Mrs Chips takes orders for the school dinners run. Telegraph.co.uk 16 September 2006. Online. Available: http://www.telegraph.co.uk/news/main.jhtml?xml=/news/2006/09/16/nmeals16.xml

6

Justice

"Justice is a habit whereby a man renders to each one his due with constant and perpetual will."

Justinian in *Corpus Iuris Civilis*

The concept of justice extends from what is done for and to the individual to include the attitudes, behaviours, policies and rules that are applied in groups, societies and nations. It is at the core of the national and international legal system and it has an important role in ethics. Justice, as one of the four classical cardinal virtues (along with temperance, courage and prudence), dates from the teachings of the philosophers of Ancient Greece and was also recognized by the Romans:

"Each man should so conduct himself that fortitude appear in labours and dangers: temperance in foregoing pleasures: prudence in the choice between good and evil: justice in giving every man his own."

Marcus Cicero in *De Officiis*

and later appears in Christian/Western doctrines. Justice means treating other people with fairness and without prejudice. It encompasses equality, impartiality and objectivity. Yet, underlying the notion of justice is the subjectivity of who decides what is just.

LEGAL JUSTICE

In law, justice is, to a large extent, prescribed. The ways in which it should be applied are written and codified in statutes and in common law. What is just in the legal sense is decided by the government and by courts. It follows long-standing traditions that have a basis in religious teaching and are grounded in morality, and is applied in a reactive way, i.e. in response to some behaviour or occurrence. The law acts 'in the interests of justice' to protect citizens from crime and exploitation, and to dispense punishments to perpetrators of criminal acts and penalties to those who are in breach of the law.

The application of justice may also vary depending on the person and the situation. This means that two people who commit the same crime or breach can be given different punishments. This may not appear to be fair. A sense of justice would surely demand that the punishment fit the crime? Yet there are a number of other factors to consider. Take the case of Terry who appears before the magistrates' court for a speeding offence. He was driving at 15 miles per hour over the speed limit in a 60 miles per hour zone. He has done this before and has been warned on many occasions. He has had past convictions for speeding and related driving offences, and has only just recovered his licence after a period of disqualification. Terry does not appear to be concerned about a speeding charge. Tim presents to the same court for the same offence. Tim has a clean driving record and has been driving for nearly 30 years. He is very remorseful and tells the court that, on the day he was speeding, he was distressed. He had received a call at work to say that his wife had collapsed and had been taken to hospital. He was in a hurry to see her but acknowledges that this is not an excuse. He is right. This will not excuse his actions but it is a mitigating factor and, taken together with his exemplary driving record, is likely to result in Tim receiving a more lenient penalty than Terry. (The exact value of a fine and the number of points that are taken for speeding are at the discretion of the court.) So, even though justice is prescribed in law, there is flexibility in the system. This allows for differences between people and situations, and it takes into account mitigating factors and valid reasons. It can (and does), however, lead to accusations of unfairness and inequality. If Terry was a manual labourer earning a basic salary and Tim a consultant neurosurgeon who earned a wage commensurate with his status, differences in penalties given by the courts could be misinterpreted as an injustice against the working class man and favouritism for the professional. However, if our legal justice system became so rigid that it did not take into account differences between people, their circumstances and a range of other relevant factors, the outcry against injustice would probably be louder.

Not only does legal justice have to deal with disparities between people and their circumstances at any given time, it also has to make temporal adjustments. Sometimes changes to the law need to be made as inequalities are exposed and challenged and to account for changes in societal views and perspectives. When considering issues of justice and fairness, changes that are made need to be done with caution and forethought about the consequences. In modern society, there is a tendency to challenge what are perceived as outdated and unfair laws or to ask for recognition of rights because a group of people feels that current laws are unjust to them.

Disability Discrimination Act – provision of services

The Disability Discrimination Act 1995 was introduced into UK law to recognize and protect the rights of the disabled. This piece of legislation forced people to look more closely at the definition of disability and to consider how much of this is caused by the norms that society has set and not by the person who may have some impairment. A good example of this is a flight of stairs. For a person who has two able legs and can walk unaided, climbing stairs is rarely considered to be problematic. Perhaps when there are several flights and fatigue starts to set in, stairs may become an inconvenience. For a person who cannot walk with ease or at all, stairs present much more than a test of fitness: they are an obstacle that can range from difficult (for an individual with a walking stick) to a complete barrier to entry (for an individual who is wheelchair bound). In the past, people who could not walk had to rely on the help of another person if stairs were the only means of approach and, more significantly, had to suffer what many felt was the indignity of being carried up the stairs. Yet, a perfectly adequate solution could have been made available: a ramp. The Disability Discrimination Act 1995 now makes it mandatory that a provider of services is under a duty to take reasonable steps to remove obstacles to entry and access (section 21(2)), and to amend practices, policies and procedures that may render the service difficult or impossible for anyone with a disability (section 21(1)).

Limitations of legal justice – the balance of individual rights against societal good

Even with the very best intentions to limit discrimination and to treat people fairly, there are occasions when groups of people feel that they and/or their lifestyle are not treated justly. Caution is sometimes advisable when attempts are made to use justice to challenge the accepted morality that underpins our laws. An extreme example of this was seen in the Netherlands in 2006, when a group of paedophiles formed a political party to campaign for the lowering and eventual abolishment of the age of consent to sexual activity (Coughlan 2006). They maintained that the current law was depriving children of their rights and unfairly criminalizing those who wish to engage in sex with young children. The move towards greater equality and justice should not overlook basic concepts of what is right and what is wrong, and should never fail to recognize that the perceived rights of an individual or small group may be at odds with what is good for society as a whole.

JUSTICE AS AN ETHICAL PRINCIPLE

Ethics, unlike law, is proactive. It does not follow a written rule or legal precedent. Justice from an ethical perspective may appear, therefore, to be less cumbersome and restrictive than legal justice because it does not include the complexities of law enforcement and protection, and does not have to follow rules and regulations. It is about treating those with whom we come into contact impartially and without prejudice. Prejudices can and should be controlled and preferably eliminated, but it may be more difficult to be impartial. There will always be people whom we like and admire and those with whom we have little in common and in whose presence we may feel uncomfortable. There will be a natural preference for some people, and this is seen from a very young age. In the school playground, children with similar interests will naturally gravitate towards one another. Liking A more than B is acceptable and is not unjust. It becomes an issue if A and B are competing for a job, award or position where partiality should have no place. If B is the better qualified, a personal preference for A is not acceptable and would not be just.

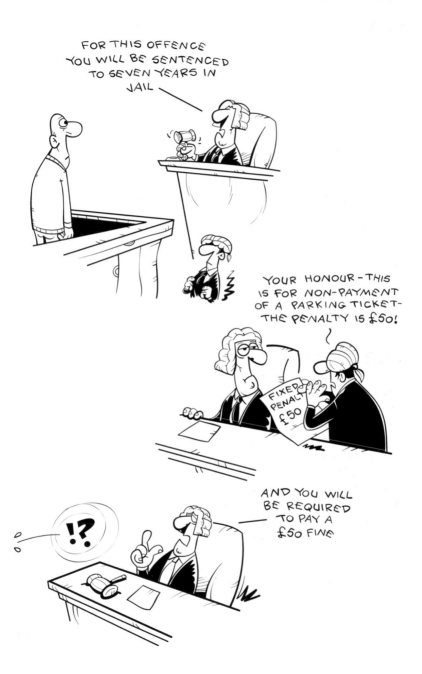

Legislation protects against discrimination on the grounds of gender, race, sexual orientation, disability, age and religious affiliation. In spite of this, discrimination on all these grounds and for a number of other reasons continues to occur. A person may be treated in an unfair way at work simply because he is clever and able and perceived to be a threat to a peer or manager. The discrimination may not obvious and may be hard to define; the person is passed over for promotion and given very difficult tasks with work performance measured according to impossibly high standards. This happens all too frequently, particularly where the working environment is highly competitive. Justice is often forgotten when people feel pressured to compete and are threatened by the performance of others who are perceived to be competitors. An ethical approach to justice needs to recognize when partiality, prejudice and personal fear may affect and distort judgement.

In a clinical context, justice means that all patients should be treated with the same respect and caring approach. This does not mean that all patients need to be given the same examination, equal time and similar advice: these will vary according to the patient and their needs. It does mean that partiality with respect to personal differences should never affect the treatment and care that is given. A practitioner may feel very strongly about a certain issue and be personally opposed to certain behaviours or practices. This ought not to be translated into a disrespectful approach towards a patient who may live his or her life according to such behaviour. For example, a practitioner may be an atheist and feel strongly that religious belief is folly. This should not have any effect on his feelings towards and consequent treatment of a priest, rabbi, imam or other patient who has clearly devoted their life to a religious faith. In practice, as in life, it can be extremely difficult at times to exercise impartiality and overlook personal characteristics in others that are at odds with our own beliefs, likes and preferences. Awareness that we are all prone to being partial and even prejudiced is most important in controlling and avoiding injustice.

JUDGEMENT

Justice has a great deal to do with judgement. In law, judgement is part of dispensing justice. In life, we make judgements about people and situations because judging situations is a necessary part of decision-making. Alternatives have to be considered and compared before any fair decision can be made. Judging people is a different matter. Sometimes it is required, as when selecting applicants for a job. The judgement in such a case is made according to pre-set criteria that determine which applicant is best suited for the job. In many other instances we have no criteria and we make our judgements against a standard that we have set for ourselves or for those to whom we are close. Perhaps the standard is one that is expected for an employee, perhaps it is for a life partner or lover, or perhaps it is a standard that we want our children to meet. If the standard is very high, the judgement may be too harsh, and the person will be judged unfairly as falling short of requirements. In judging others we need to be sure that the standards against which the judgement is made are fair for that particular person. If the receptionist at your practice is taking a little longer obtaining basic details from patients than the receptionist she replaced, it may be because she is new to the job and requires some time to learn to work to speed. It could also be that she naturally takes longer with people because she likes to chat to them and make them feel comfortable. In the long run this could help with your practice. Unless she is neglecting fundamental aspects of her job, it would not be fair to expect her to work in exactly the same way as did the previous receptionist.

Information needed to make a judgement

In addition to a standard against which situations or people are judged, judgements also require information. For a sound judgement to be made, information must be accurate and sufficient. Sometimes it may appear as though a situation is clear and obvious, and yet a vital piece of information, which could alter the judgement entirely, is missing.

The woman on the radio

On a late night radio programme a panel of experts were taking calls from and offering advice to members of the public about marital and family problems A woman called the panel and explained that she had a very happy marriage and 2 years ago had given birth to a healthy and beautiful baby boy. The problem was that she now wanted a second child but her husband was against it. This was the only point on which the two of them had ever

Continued

disagreed and she did not want this to create a rift between them. She did, however, really wish to have another baby. The panel members were very sympathetic to the woman and offered her a number of solutions and methods that she may try in order to convince her husband to agree to another child. After a short lull in the conversation, one member of the panel asked the woman the following question:

'How old are you?'

'Twenty-one', she answered.

'And how old is your husband?'

There was a slight hesitation…:' Seventy-one'.

There was a stunned silence. Then a panel member coughed and cleared his throat. Slowly, one by one, the panel members spoke, this time cautiously advising the woman about the need to understand her husband and his point of view, on the joys of having a single child and on the importance of maintaining a happy marriage.

The initial advice was completely altered. The panel had misjudged the situation and the husband's motives, because they had made their judgements without a very simple but crucial piece of information.

(Panel discussion heard by the author in Melbourne, Australia.)

Collecting the right information is crucial in clinical practice, for diagnosis, for understanding the needs and wishes of the patient, and for proper treatment. For a fair and just diagnosis, the practitioner is reliant on the patient reporting symptoms fully. It is also important to ascertain how a condition may be affecting or restricting the way in which the patient needs to function at work, at home and in other daily activities. If the patient does not report the true or full extent of symptoms, the practitioner will find it difficult to make a fair and just assessment. Patients who have disturbing symptoms can become very fearful that the symptoms may be an indication that their sight is becoming impaired. Such a patient may come into the practice too scared to reveal the full extent of symptoms for fear of hearing that they have a debilitating and sight-threatening condition. The patient may skirt around the symptom, hoping that some other piece of information will prompt the practitioner to tell them that there is nothing seriously wrong. A practitioner may feel that they are not being told the full truth and wrongly conclude that the patient is being obstructive or perhaps malingering. This diagnosis would not be correct but could be understandable given that the patient has not been totally honest or fair to the practitioner.

Just as justice requires all the facts for a fair judgment, clinical diagnosis requires an honest description of symptoms. In the clinical situation, the practitioner is always in the more powerful position. In order to be fair and just, it may at times require a greater effort to extract the pertinent information from a patient whose lack of openness stems from fear and not from deliberate obstruction or unjustified distrust.

Clinical case study

Maria comes to see you, complaining that the reading glasses that you pre-scribed for her are not 'good enough'. You are puzzled about this because they were dispensed only 3 weeks ago to replace a pair that she had broken. The original (broken) pair had only been prescribed 6 months earlier. Maria seems distracted and complains about headaches and things 'swimming around'. You check the spectacle power and the fitting of the frame and find no errors. Distance and near acuity have not changed since the original prescription was given. Maria keeps insisting that it must be these glasses because she had no problems with previous spectacles.

You are starting to get a little frustrated as you have taken Maria in at very short notice and you have had a very busy and stressful day. You are about to give up and tell Maria to persevere for another week, but decide to do an ophthalmoscopic examination to confirm what you suspect: that Maria is malingering. In the right eye you see a large vitreous floater. There is no retinal tear. You question Maria further and find that the things she said were 'swimming around' refer to the floater. On further probing she ventures that she sees 'shiny speckles and stars' sometimes. They seem to her to be more noticeable when she is reading and that is why blames the glasses. Maria has had a posterior vitreous detachment. There is no retinal tear but you refer her to an ophthalmologist and inform her that she will need to come in for examinations every 6 months. Maria is reassured that there is no damage to her eye and she then opens up and admits how frightened she was that she might be going blind.

Trust in the judgement

Once a decision has been made based on evaluation of the appro-priate information and sound judgement, that decision should be trusted by the person to whom it will apply. When a practitioner takes a case history, conducts a clinical examination, analyses the information collected and evaluates options, these will be presented to the patient. The patient needs to be able to trust that they have received a thorough examination and fair and sound evaluation of the treatment or further tests needed for the condition. If a patient does not trust the clinical judgement of a practitioner, the application of justice is hampered.

There may be a number of reasons why trust is missing in a practitioner–patient relationship. There may have been a history of errors made in examinations in the past, either with that practitioner or with others. Perhaps the practitioner has not always told the patient all details of a condition and the patient has discovered this through another source. This can frequently occur when a practitioner observes changes that pose no immediate threat to vision, such as early-stage opacification in the lens. The practitioner sees no reason to mention this to the patient because there is no action that needs to be taken, and he considers it unnecessary to alarm the patient. Within a year the patient has cause to come in for another eye examination. This time another practitioner sees the patient. This practitioner mentions the lens opacities. The patient becomes doubtful about the clinical skills and judgement of the first practitioner. The seeds of doubt will remain and the necessary trust between patient and practitioner will be compromised.

A relationship of trust may also be missing when a practitioner sees a new patient. Time is needed to build up such a relationship, and some patients may need more time than others. A lack of trust may also be based on fear. If a patient has a condition that is sight-threatening, the trust in the practitioner and his or her judgement is even more crucial than it may be if the outcome is simply a change in spectacle prescription. When the risk to sight is greater, the need for trust in the practitioner is ever more important. Yet, sometimes that is precisely when a lack of trust becomes evident, because the patient may want assurance that sight will not be lost and the practitioner may be unable to give that assurance. There may be uncertainty in the prognosis and uncertainty in treatment outcomes. A patient may misinterpret the uncertainty as the practitioner being reluctant to divulge bad news. In such a situation, patience and honesty, as well as empathy for the patient and their situation, are needed to help the patient find trust in the practitioner and the clinical judgement. It may require recommending that the patient obtain a second opinion. A second opinion should not be seen as reinforcing the distrust of the patient in the abilities of the practitioner, but as a way of reassuring the patient that the practitioner is sure of their judgement and does not mind it being compared with that of another practitioner.

Trust in any relationship should be mutual. In healthcare practice, where the patient is in the vulnerable position, the practitioner needs to remember that greater effort needs to be made in order to earn and retain the trust of the patient. This is particularly important with a new or fearful patient.

DISTRIBUTIVE JUSTICE

Justice in society also applies to resources and their distribution. The concept of distributive justice can be traced back to Aristotle, who made a distinction between justice as provided by the law and that which applies to fairness in actions of people towards other people (Rescher 1967). This second type of justice Aristotle subcategorized into 'corrective' and 'distributive' justice. *Corrective justice* describes the fairness with which an individual treats others; *distributive justice* is about the equitable behaviour of the state in the way it distributes resources (Rescher 1967). Before deciding how to allocate resources it is important to determine the basis or the 'canon of justice' on which the distribution will be made (Rescher 1967). Rescher describes seven canons of distributive justice:

1. Resources should be distributed equally to all.
2. Resources should be distributed according to need.
3. Resources should be distributed according to merit or achievement.
4. Resources should be distributed according to effort and sacrifice.
5. Resources should be distributed according to productivity.
6. Resources should be distributed according to the public interest or greater good.
7. Resources should be distributed according to socially useful services or supply scarcity.

All are forms of distributive justice and each is contentious and problematic. When applied to health care, distribution of resources according to one or other of the canons solely will result in some measure of injustice.

Distributing resources equally to all

This would appear to be the fairest distribution because it makes no judgement about the patient. Yet it also fails to distinguish between patients with greater and lesser needs and unequal claims to health care. The presbyope who needs reading glasses occasionally does not require the same resource allocation in terms of consultation time, dispensing and aftercare as the disabled elderly patient with low vision who needs more time to communicate her needs, to be examined and to be allowed to select the appropriate low vision aid. To determine that each patient will receive the same level of resources will result in an injustice to most: some will be given more resources than they need or want, and others will receive too little time and effort. Equal resource allocation overlooks the basic fact that not all people behave in the same way, need the same examinations, or can afford the same treatment.

Distributing resources according to need

Healthcare provision according to the needs that a patient has may seem to be fair. Whether or not a person can afford to pay for treatment should have no bearing on the treatment received. This system would work if resources were aplenty and the society served by this system was relatively unchanging in the way its needs were distributed, so that needs and resources could be well matched. There is no such model society. Even in the developed world, healthcare resources cannot always match demand. Certain debilitating and life-threatening diseases (such as smallpox and polio) that have been eradicated in the developed world have been replaced by other illnesses and chronic conditions. In addition, as we have learnt to control and manage certain ailments, we have also increased life expectancy. Control and management of many conditions has not, however, led to cures. This means that more people can expect to live longer, but some may live with chronic conditions that require regular health care. Ageing itself is a risk factor for many diseases. In addition to this, the developed world faces a crisis in the health of the young. The incidence of obesity is rising and appearing at younger ages. Obesity is not an illness, but it increases the risk of many chronic conditions, such as diabetes, cardiovascular disease and arthritis. The rise in the need for healthcare provision without a concomitant rise in resources means that needs have to be classified in some way. Who should determine what sort of healthcare need is greatest and on what basis? The needs of a patient with chronic and debilitating arthritis cannot easily be compared and quantified against the needs of a patient who has lost the use of their lower limbs in an accident.

The distribution of health care according to needs has become more complicated as technology has advanced. There are now means of keeping alive babies born in the second trimester of pregnancy. In the days before such means existed, these infants died because their organs were not sufficiently developed to keep them alive without assistance. Whilst preserving life should be of paramount importance, the fragile lives that can now be extended have added to the medical needs in society and to the costs – not just as measured in monetary terms. In the case of Charlotte Wyatt, to whom reference was made in Chapter 1, the struggle of her parents (to prevent doctors from ceasing to resuscitate her whenever necessary) contributed to a breakdown in their marriage (Yeoman 2006). By her third birthday, neither parent felt able to cope with taking care of the little girl. She was left to the local hospital Trust until suitable foster care could be arranged. Given the severity of her condition – serious damage to lungs, kidney and brain – she requires expensive equipment to help her breathe and feed. The cost of keeping Charlotte alive is estimated to be £300 a day, and over the first 3 years of her life has cost more than a million pounds (Yeoman 2006). The question of whether the limited resources of the National Health Service would have been better spent on other patients, rather than on supporting the needs of a little girl who has been kept alive by artificial means, has been asked. This is a very difficult question to answer, unless one believes that a value can be placed on life and that such value is related to the fragility or perceived quality of the life.

Distributing resources according to merit or achievement, or to effort and sacrifice

Distribution according to a person's merits or efforts recognizes differences in the way that people are valued; this is linked, in our society, to what people are paid. In society it is accepted that, if a person works, they receive remuneration for their efforts. There is a right to be paid for doing a job. Salaries and wages vary enormously. Salary earned is dependent, to a large extent, on the job or occupation, and anyone in a given job or occupation has the right to earn the salary commensurate with that post. It follows, therefore, that some people earn more than others and are recognized as having a right to do so. There are a number of other rights that our society accepts as fundamental and that give rise to differentials. One of these is the right to own property, with no restrictions on amount. Some people earn a lot of money and, as they have the right to spend their money as they choose, can own many properties. Others earn a great deal less and may not be able to afford a buy a single property. The canon of 'each according to his or her merits or achievements' causes differences in wealth distribution.

In societies that have open markets and in which individuals are not restricted in what they can earn and on what that money can be spent, there will be inequalities in wealth that will have an effect on health care. Even when health care is subsidized by the state, the option of private care is available. This means that those who can afford it have the right to go to a doctor of their choice, to be spared a long wait for surgery, and to be able to pay for some treatments that may be expensive. In countries where private health care prevails, these differences in the provision of health care between the more affluent and the poorer members of society are felt even more acutely. Justice according to the patient's affordability may seem fair to those who can fully exercise their rights and can afford to pay for a wider range of treatments. It may not appear to be so fair for those who are restricted in what they can afford. In an eye care clinic there will be a range of spectacle frames of various prices and in various styles. Patients who can afford more expensive frames have a greater choice than patients with a limited budget, who may be able to select only from amongst the lower priced frames. There cannot be equality in the selection because each patient chooses according to what he or she can afford and in accordance with their rights to do so.

The inequalities and potential injustice that may be the consequence of distributing resources in accordance with a perceived achievement, effort and therefore affordability becomes even more evident when the picture is global. The developing world faces crisis after crisis with poverty, war and sickness rampant. Is it fair to say that people living in these countries should be provided only the health care that they can afford (which would equate to nothing)?

Distributing resources according to productivity

There may be some validity in arguing that an elderly pensioner who has worked hard all their life and paid taxes deserves greater access to health care in old age than one who has never made any effort to find employment, squandered what they had and has contributed little, in terms of work and paying taxes, to society. With regard to health care, the productive contribution could also be the contribution an individual makes to the maintenance of their own good health, and this would also be for the benefit of society.

If the argument for this canon is advanced with regard to health care, it would mean greater resources to those who have contributed to society through their work and their healthy lifestyle. Chronic conditions brought on by lifestyle choices, such as smoking and over-eating, are conditions that can be controlled, and even eliminated. It could be argued that, if a person chooses to engage in an unhealthy lifestyle in spite of warnings and efforts to help promote change, that person should be held responsible for any resulting illness suffered. Following this argument, when resources are limited such a person should not be the first whose needs are met. Should the needs of an obese diabetic who continues to smoke come before the patient who has cancer despite living in accordance with what is recommended for a healthy lifestyle? The difficulty with treating the patient who has no responsibility for their illness in preference to one whose lifestyle has contributed to ill-health is that healthcare provision would become a type of reward or payment for good behaviour. The consequences of such a system of distributive justice would be that those who do not work and do not have a healthy lifestyle would be denied help. These are often the poorest members of society. They may be unemployed because they have not had the opportunities for education and training. They may consume cheap and unhealthy food because they may have limited access to healthy lifestyle choices. To put these individuals at the back of the 'healthcare queue' would serve to maintain and exacerbate poor health in already deprived socioeconomic groups. This would not accord with natural justice or provide a fair distribution of resources.

Distributing resources according to public interest or the greater good for a greater number

Distributing resources to benefit the greatest number of people requires defining the 'greater good'. If it is predicated on numbers of people alone, then a greater share of global resources should go to more populated countries, even if some of these are already more affluent than some poorer nations. Within countries, differences in wealth and healthcare provision also exist. The more populated regions in the south of England could claim a greater share of healthcare resources than the less populated and generally less affluent northern regions. This would not be a just allocation. It is also one that does not take into account the future consequences of serving what may appear to be the greater good today. Restricting resources to those who are already deprived would emphasize and expand the divisions between those who have and those who do not have decent health care. This cannot serve the public interest in the long term.

Distributing resources according to usefulness in society or supply scarcity

This allocation of resources takes into account the economic formula of supply and demand. Those who are perceived to be more useful than other individuals because what they offer is rare or scarce should, according to this principle of distributive justice, be valued and allocated a greater share of resources. If this were to be applied in health care, it would require defining which groups of individuals were more socially useful than others and then deciding how much more useful they were in order to allocate to them their greater share.

The difficulty with this canon is in the determination of usefulness and whether this is a true evaluation of needs or whether it reflects a desire for the particular service. Rescher (1967) points out that, under this form of distributive justice, entertainers should receive greater pay than successful doctors. This does indeed happen, although it is debatable whether this occurs because of the relative scarcity of entertainers or whether it reflects the apparent societal value placed on fame and celebrity. However, translating such an allocation of resources to health care would not be just. It would ignore need for treatment and would be felt most acutely amongst certain socioeconomic groups and would, like the canon of distribution according to productivity, ultimately favour the more specialized and the more educated.

There may be isolated instances when legitimate argument for this canon could be advanced. If there were an outbreak of a serious pandemic that could potentially result in fatalities, and immunization was available but scarce, it could be argued that doctors and healthcare workers should be immunized before others because their services would be in greater demand.

The case of Mark Dalton

Mark Dalton worked in the laboratory of a chemical plant as a technician. His work record was excellent. One day he became ill with a renal disease and was unable to continue in his old job because it was considered by the company that the exposure to chemicals would be detrimental to his health. The company allocated him to a different post on the same salary level. However, two other people working in the company had both sought to be promoted to this post. One of these employees was female. Both of them had been trained for the position and were senior to Mark.

Each of these three people had a valid claim to the post under different principles of justice. Mark had worked hard for the company and, now that he had contracted a chronic illness, he could claim that he was entitled to recognition of his efforts and to a job with a salary equal to that of his last post. The other two employees could claim a higher level of training and therefore better suitability for the post on the grounds of merit as well as effort and contribution. The woman could also cite equal opportunity as a basis for her claim. Measures to promote equality in the workplace must take into account any gender imbalance. (Case reported by R E Stevenson and cited by Beauchamp & Childress 2001.)

In practice, resources are distributed in accordance with more than one of the canons. There is a right to basic health care for every person living in the United Kingdom, but those who can afford private care may not have to wait as long and may have their own choice of practitioner. In addition, the more affluent and better educated will be more aware and have greater access to products, treatment and methods available for the maintenance of good health.

Globally there is recognition that every human being should have adequate health care:

"Everyone has the right to a standard of living adequate for the health and wellbeing of himself and of his family, including housing and medical care and necessary social services."

United Nations Universal Declaration of Human Rights
1948, Article 25(1)

This is fine and noble and, if it could be achieved, there would be no reason to disagree with the basic tenet. The problem is that it is difficult to achieve. The glaring discrepancy between living standards in the developed and the developing world attests to that.

Even within developed countries there are large differences in the living standards of the wealthy and the poor. The declaration does not take into account how this right is to be met, nor does it explain what is meant by adequate. If 'adequate' requires more resources than are available, then clearly it cannot be met. Alternatively, adequate could be defined as the amount that is available to each person once resources had been fairly and justly distributed. This leads back to deciding the basis on which this distribution should be made.

SUMMARY

Justice in clinical practice needs to take account of the legalities of justice as well as the ethical aspects. All patients deserve the basic standard of care that is prescribed by law, avoiding any form of discrimination. The practitioner should be aware that, although patients will present with differing needs and expectations, and will make different choices, they deserve to be treated with a fair and just approach. Resource allocation has no basis that can be just to all.

References

Beauchamp T L, Childress J F 2001 Principles of biomedical ethics, 5th edn. Oxford University Press, New York, p 229

Coughlan G 2006 Dutch alarmed by paedophile group. BBC News 1 June 2006. Online. Available: http://news.bbc.co.uk/2/hi/europe/5038682.stm

Disability Discrimination Act 1995 Offi ce of Public Sector Information. Online. Available: http://www.opsi.gov.uk/acts/acts1995/Ukpga_19950050_en_1.htm

Rescher N 1967 Distributive justice. Bobbs-Merrill, Indianapolis University Press of America

United Nations Universal Declaration of Human Rights 1948. Online. Available: http://www.un.org/Overview/rights.html

Yeoman F 2006 Carers sought for baby Charlotte as parents part. Times-Online 17 October 2006. Online. Available: http://www.timesonline.co.uk/tol/news/uk/health/article602823.ece

7

Confidentiality/ data protection

The principle of confidentiality has an ethical and a legal basis, and sometimes the two appear to conflict. If there is such a conflict, the law will prevail. This can give the mistaken impression that confidentiality is a legal concept that is strictly regulated and as such leaves little to the discretion of the practitioner. In healthcare practice, as in many other aspects of life, there are situations concerning confidentiality that the law does not cover. In such cases, the decision to disclose personal information needs to be made on the basis of the personal ethics of the individual practitioner.

CONFIDENTIALITY AS AN ETHICAL CONCEPT

The preservation of and respect for confidentiality in health care dates back to the Hippocratic Oath:

"Whatever I see or hear, professionally or privately, which ought not to be divulged, I will keep secret and tell no one."

Modern medicine and health care applies the principles of confidentiality to all of these aspects of interaction between the practitioner and the patient.

The respect for confidences and secrets is a fundamental respect for another person and what he or she holds to be intimate or private. There is a paradoxical need in people to protect privacy and preserve intimacy, and yet at the same time to fulfil the desire to share some aspect of this intimacy with another. This develops early in life. Young children in primary school tell secrets to their friends. The sharing of a secret between two people seals a bond of trust between them. The one who tells the secret and the one to whom the secret is told both understand that they share privileged and intimate information, and often there is a mutual sharing of secrets. When one person reveals, to a third party, intimate information that they had promised to keep, trust has been betrayed and the bonds of friendship may be severed. This can, depending on the nature of the relationship and the information divulged, cause total and irreversible breakdown in the relationship. Indeed, often when a person is deemed not to be trustworthy, it is not because they have committed some crime or distrustful act, but rather that they have been unable or unwilling to protect and respect secrets or intimate information.

The principle of confidentiality relies on trust: trust in the judgement, maturity, wisdom and above all integrity of the one to whom secret or private details are revealed. In healthcare practice, trust underpins the relationship between the practitioner and the patient. The patient puts their trust in the expertise and knowledge of the practitioner; the patient also trusts the practitioner to protect whatever personal data and information the practitioner has about them. This information may extend beyond what is related to the patient's ocular or general health. The patient may trust the practitioner with personal information. This can be because the patient and practitioner have known each other for years and the patient feels at ease sharing personal information. It may also be for the very opposite reason: because the practitioner is a stranger, and sometimes very personal matters are easier to share with a stranger, especially one who is in a position of trust.

Keeping information and data confidential is a form of protection for both the person and the information that he or she has provided. There are times, however, when protecting the information could actually harm the individual who has revealed it, or could cause danger to others. In some of these instances, the law obliges the practitioner to breach confidentiality. At other times, the decision rests with the practitioner to determine whether the information or the person should be protected.

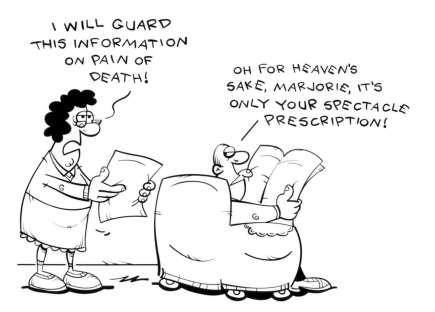

Protecting the secret or the protecting the person?

There may be occasions when the practitioner is asked by a patient to keep confidential information that the practitioner feels would be in the interests of the patient to reveal. This does not include information that is required to be disclosed by law (covered later), for what must be disclosed under the law is more prescriptive and does not leave the choice of disclosure with the practitioner. In a situation where there is no legal requirement to reveal confidential information and the patient has requested that the information remain undisclosed, but keeping the information in confidence may be a risk to the patient, a practitioner has no guidelines and has to make a decision in accordance with his or her own ethical perspective and reasoning. Such decisions can arise when the patient is in a difficult and even dangerous situation in which the choices that are made are based on fear: the patient fears that revealing the information will bring them more harm than keeping the information secret. Such a patient is extremely vulnerable and, whatever the practitioner decides, the vulnerability of the patient and the consequences of the decision to disclose or not to disclose must be considered very carefully.

Protecting the vulnerable adult

To some extent, all patients are vulnerable because the patient comes to the practitioner for help. The degree of vulnerability varies and some patients are more vulnerable than others. Young children, frail or elderly adults, and those who may be disabled or incapacitated in a way that can affect their decision-making and understanding, are more vulnerable than an autonomous adult patient who does not have a disability.

The College of Optometrists has listed, as vulnerable patients, children and adults who have physical disabilities, substantial learning difficulties, are physically or mentally ill, are impaired because of alcohol, substance abuse or because of advanced age (College of Optometrists 2007, Code of Ethics, Section 26). These patients require greater protection and, because of this, their confidentiality may, at times, need to be given particularly careful consideration.

Clinical case study

An elderly woman comes into your practice and she is clearly distressed. Her case history and examination show that there is nothing wrong with her eyes. You sense that something else is bothering her and you ask her whether she would like to talk. After a further period of procrastination, the patient breaks down, starts to cry, and lifts up the sleeves of her blouse to reveal large black bruises along her arm. You express great concern and prompt her to tell you more. She reveals that she is often beaten up by her son, who is on drugs and who regularly demands money from her.

You tell her that she should report this to the police immediately, but she looks horrified. 'I can't report my son to the police. I don't want to get him into any trouble.'
She looks at you with tears in her eyes and pleads: 'Please don't tell anyone about this'.

What would you do?
(Based on a situation the author faced in clinical practice.)

In the above situation it is clear that whichever decision is taken – to report the situation or to keep the requested confidence – some pain and distress will be caused to the patient. As the matter is not one that has anything to do with the patient's sight or visual needs, it will not appear on the record card and no other practitioner will see it. The woman is no danger to any other person, and therefore there is no requirement by law to report her. Any danger that does exist is that to the woman herself. Nevertheless, as an autonomous and competent adult she has asked that the information she has shared with the practitioner remain 'secret'. The reasons for this are complex and deeply emotional, because they involve the love of a mother for her child and the instinctive need to protect him. There may also be an underlying feeling of shame that she has failed as a parent and the unrelenting hope that her son will one day recover. If the matter was reported, the victim could (and probably would) deny any knowledge of the abuse. Indeed, this frequently happens in cases of domestic violence. If the practitioner did go against the wishes of the patient and report the matter, the patient may well feel that her trust in the practitioner had been betrayed and that her confidence had not been protected. However, the practitioner may consider that in this case the woman herself needs protecting. She is the victim of a crime and at risk of further and greater harm. The decision depends on what is perceived to be the least painful consequence, and what and who is in greatest need of protection: the woman or her secret (and her son).

Protecting the patient from self-harm and harm to others

Clinical case study

A 26-year-old man comes to your practice saying that he would like to try contact lenses. He has been wearing spectacles with a low spherical prescription and tells you that sometimes he finds glasses cumbersome, especially when playing sport and driving. No contraindications to contact lens wear are found and the patient reports no discomfort with lens fitting.
A trial set is given to the patient to see how he will adapt to contact lens wear. A week later he returns saying that he has had no discomfort and that he will now be wearing contact lenses instead of spectacles all the time. Whilst you are making some notes, the patient expresses again his enthusiasm for contact lenses and adds that he was getting a little worried about wearing spectacles because when he has an epileptic fit they sometimes fall off and could break. You ask the patient whether he holds a full driving

Continued

licence, and he answers that he does. You inform him that he can be permitted to drive only if he has not had an epileptic seizure for at least a year, and that if he has a seizure it is his responsibility to contact the appropriate authority and to surrender his licence or he will be breaking the law. The patient immediately replies that it has been a long time since he has had a fit and that it has probably been somewhat longer than a year.

You do not have the name of the patient's GP on the record card and ask whether he could give you this information. The patient replies that he has recently moved and has not registered with a local practice. He says that he does not remember the name or address of his last GP.

The responsibility of informing the appropriate driving licensing authority about epilepsy rests with the individual. If the affected individual neglects to do this, the doctor, or any healthcare practitioner, is legally bound to report the matter to the appropriate driving authority in order to protect the public. However, in this case, the practitioner does not have all of the necessary information about this patient and his condition. He or she cannot, therefore, be sure when the patient last had an epileptic seizure and whether reporting is indeed necessary. The patient may be telling the truth about not having had a seizure for over a year. To report the matter would be likely to cause the patient to feel not only that the practitioner could not be trusted but also to experience a sense of being slighted. The practitioner has not trusted him when he said that he had not had a seizure for over a year. To report the matter does indeed indicate that the patient is not being trusted to tell the truth. This may be justified, and potential accidents and dangers averted.

A preferred course of action would have been to inform the patient's GP, who should have the pertinent information and be able to say whether or not the patient has been seizure-free for over a year. If not, the patient should be notified that, if he does not inform the appropriate authority, the practitioner will be obliged to do so. However, in this case the patient is not able to or does not wish to divulge the contact details of his GP. Perhaps, the patient would respond positively to a gentle reminder that, if the GP details are not provided, the practitioner will have to notify the appropriate authority because there is uncertainty over the risk of a seizure. This may prompt the patient to find and reveal the contact details of his GP. Conversely, such a reminder may indicate to the patient that there is a lack of trust in him, and this may alienate and upset the patient.

Any further information may then be refused. The decision to report the matter in such a case will ultimately rest with the practitioner, who needs to consider that any reporting will be breaching confidentiality. It may turn out that there was no reason to do so, if the patient was telling the truth. This has to be balanced against the possibility of a real risk to the patient and his passengers, other drivers and pedestrians if the patient is hiding the facts for fear of losing his licence. The practitioner has a duty to protect the public before the duty to protect the confidentiality of any individual patient.

Protecting children

Children are a particularly vulnerable group of patients. They rely on decisions made for them by parents, guardians and carers, and society entrusts these people with responsibility for children. Unfortunately, there are cases in which this trust is betrayed. Young children who are abused, either physically or mentally, by a parent or legal guardian are often unable to complain about the abuse or know to whom or how to report the abuser. They, as any victim of abuse, will be frightened of the abuser and the element of fear will frequently prevent the victim from speaking out or admitting, when questioned, that abuse has occurred.

Clinical case study

A 5-year old girl is referred to you by the school. The referral letter cites poor concentration and suspected difficulties with seeing the board as the reason for referral. The child comes to see you accompanied by her mother. As she sits on the chair, you cannot help but notice bruises on her arms and legs. Looking closer, you see what look like two cigarette burns on the inside of her right arm. You ask the mother about the bruising and the marks, and she replies that the child is very active but is often quite careless and has consequently had many minor accidents. She goes on to say that the burns were indeed caused by cigarettes and this happened because the child had rushed into her father's arms before he had had a chance to extinguish a cigarette that he was smoking at the time.

Examining the child, you take extra care to look for any signs that may suggest abuse but, beyond the bruising and the burn marks, the examination reveals nothing extraordinary that may fuel added suspicion of abuse.

Do you make a note of what you have observed but not take the matter any further? There is a chance that the mother is telling the truth; she has an unruly youngster to handle and reporting this parent to social services would only cause her unnecessary distress. Or do you take the risk of reporting a potentially innocent parent because you consider that the risk of so doing is far outweighed by the risk of leaving a vulnerable child exposed to further abuse? A decision in such a situation is extremely difficult.

If a practitioner genuinely suspects a case of child abuse, there is an ethical expectation to submit this information to an appropriate authority because reporting is an act of protecting a patient, especially one who is particularly vulnerable, from further harm. In recent times, the ethical expectation has become more of an obligation, as prominent cases of child abuse reported in the media have highlighted, to medical and healthcare professions as well as to social services and other relevant authorities, the consequences of not reporting. After the tragic case of Victoria Climbié, healthcare practitioners and others who come into contact with children are expected to be more vigilant and are encouraged to report suspected instances of abuse, even if this breaches confidentiality.

The case of Victoria Climbié

Victoria Climbié was born in the Ivory Coast and brought to Europe by Marie-Thérèse Kouao, an aunt of her father. It is understood that the arrangement was made between Victoria's parents and the father's aunt in order to give Victoria educational and other opportunities she may not have had in the Ivory Coast. When she left her home and family, Victoria was 7 years old, a happy, healthy and intelligent child. The original arrangement was for Marie-Thérèse to take Victoria to France, and Victoria did spend 5 months in France before Marie-Thérèse brought her to the United Kingdom in April 1999.

On 14 June of the same year, a distant acquaintance of Marie-Thérèse noticed a scar on the little girl's cheek. The child's body was covered with clothing so that her arms and legs were not visible. When Mrs Ackah, the acquaintance, asked about this, Marie-Thérèse said that Victoria had fallen on an escalator. Mrs Ackah, however, was sufficiently concerned, as she had noted that, since she first met Victoria at the end of April to the time she noted the scar in mid June, the little girl had lost weight and looked frail. She reported

Continued

the matter to the social services in Ealing on 18 June 1999. Staff at the social services had noticed the forlorn appearance of the child in May. It is notable that a nurse at a GP surgery where Victoria was seen on 8 June 1999 did not examine her physically and did not appear to be sufficiently observant to note the child's gaunt physical appearance. Neither the nurse nor social services staff did anything, at that point, to investigate the matter further.

Around mid June 1999, Marie-Thérèse met Carl Manning, who very soon after became her lover. Victoria was put into the daily care of an experienced childminder, who was not registered. This woman, who looked after Victoria from 7 a.m. until late evening, because Marie-Thérèse was working, treated the little girl well, but noted Marie-Thérèse's harshness towards the child and Victoria's fear of her aunt. She also noted signs of physical abuse. Marie-Thérèse always had an explanation for any marks or bruises.

On 13 July, Marie-Thérèse brought Victoria to the childminder, asking her to take the child for good because Manning did not want her living with them. The childminder agreed to take Victoria for one night only, and it was on that night that she noted signs of severe abuse: burns, bruising, loose skin, facial swelling and fingers oozing pus. The next day, the childminder took Victoria to the accident and emergency department of the Middlesex Hospital, where the examining physician became very concerned about potential abuse and referred the child to a paediatric registrar. The registrar also agreed that some of the injuries may not be accidental, and the police were called. Victoria was placed under police protection. Marie-Thérèse found out about this and arrived at the hospital as Victoria was being seen by the doctor conducting the ward round. This doctor provided an incorrect diagnosis of scabies that resulted in Victoria being put into isolation, given the highly infectious nature of the disease. By the next morning, the police withdrew their protection, as the earlier diagnosis of abuse had now been overtaken by one of scabies, and Victoria was returned to her aunt.

A week later, Victoria returned to hospital suffering from serious facial scalding. Marie-Thérèse explained that this was caused by Victoria putting her head under the hot water tap as she tried to relieve the itchiness caused by scabies. Victoria stayed in hospital for almost 2 weeks, and during that time a number of medical staff noted signs of serious abuse. They also noted the fear the child had of Marie-Thérèse and Carl Manning when they came to visit.

Victoria was released from hospital back to the care of Marie-Thérèse. The social worker assigned to her case visited her at home 10 days later and found her well dressed and apparently in good care. The social worker asked no questions about schooling and did not speak to the child. Subsequent

Continued

visits from the social worker did not elicit any alarming reports and it appears that Victoria was cleaned and told how to behave before visits by the social worker. Allegations made by Marie-Thérèse, in November 1999, of sexual abuse of Victoria by Manning, which were later withdrawn, did not prompt detailed investigation.

For a further 4 months Victoria continued to live with her abusers and the treatment she received at their hands became progressively worse. Towards the end of her life, she was locked in the bathroom, tied up in a plastic sack, left to lie in her own excrement, her hands and feet bound by masking tape – she was forced to eat like a domestic animal. She suffered beatings with shoes, hammers, coat hangers and other implements. After months of abuse, Victoria was admitted to hospital with severe hypothermia and organ failure. Shortly after arrival, she suffered respiratory and cardiac arrest. Staff were unable to save her and, on 25 February 2000, Victoria Climbié died aged 8 years and 3 months. (Based on the official report by Lord Laming, Department of Health 2003)

The sequence of events that resulted in the death of Victoria Climbié indicated a number of instances where intervention by healthcare and other authorities could and ought to have been made. Although concerns were raised, the word of the carer, Marie-Thérèse, appeared to be paramount, and confidentiality, in this case erroneously, was preserved. The child was entrusted to the carer and appropriate checks were not made to see whether the carer was worthy of this trust. It is always difficult to interfere in what are perceived to be domestic and therefore private, family matters.

In our society there is an implicit trust in parents, guardians and carers, for they are held to be more reliable than those who depend on their care. To question the parent, guardian or carer is not easy and reporting them requires a breach of confidence. It may also result in suspicion being placed on an innocent person and this has to be carefully weighed against the decision to leave a child at risk of abuse or even more serious consequences. In situations where there is uncertainty about whether or not abuse may be taking place, the practitioner needs to be prepared to make a very difficult decision with little formal guidance.

CONFIDENTIALITY IN LAW

Confidentiality has some protection in law. There is a general legal obligation not to disclose information that may identify a person. This applies not only to healthcare professionals dealing with patients but to any person or organization that holds personal details about an individual.

Data Protection Act 1998

The Data Protection Act 1998 provides people with legally enforceable rights with respect to their personal data or any information that can provide a means of identification. It offers a way of protecting and respecting the privacy of individuals. A practitioner in any area of health care deals with a great deal of personal information, primarily with respect to patients but also with respect to employees.

The Data Protection Act 1998 describes the information that needs to be kept confidential and defines two categories of data that must be protected: personal data (section 1(1)) and sensitive personal data (section 2)).

'Personal data' are those that relate to a living individual and that either provide a means of identifying that person or that, together with other information held by the practitioner, can provide a means of identifying the person. This includes such information as name, contact details and date of birth. It is notable that the definition includes 'expressions of opinion', and any suggestion of the data controller's (practitioner's) intentions in respect of the person (section 1(1)). The Act does not clarify the nature of opinions or intentions.

'Sensitive personal data' are particularly relevant to healthcare practice because they cover information about the physical and/or mental health of an individual (section 2(e)). This also includes information about race or ethnic origin (s2(a)), political opinions (s2(b)) and religious beliefs (s2(c)).

Unauthorized disclosure of personal or sensitive personal data is punishable by a fine (s60). The professional body may well impose a further penalty on a practitioner convicted under the Data Protection Act.

The Data Protection principles

The Data Protection Act is based on eight principles, known as the principles of 'good information handling' (Schedule 1, Part1, Data Protection Act 1998).

These eight principles, which must be followed when handling personal and sensitive personal data, state that such data must be:

1. fairly and lawfully processed;
2. obtained for lawful and specified purposes and processed for those purposes;
3. adequate, relevant and not excessive;
4. accurate and up to date;
5. not kept longer than necessary (this is determined by the data controller – the practitioner);
6. processed in accordance with the data subject's rights as specified in the Act;
7. secure – appropriate technical and organizational measures must be taken to protect against unauthorized or unlawful processing of personal data and against accidental loss or destruction of personal data;
8. not transferred to countries outside the European Economic Area that are without adequate protection for processing of personal data.

Handling of personal data

Data are handled primarily by the data controller, the practitioner, and can be accessible to a restricted group of other people. Accessibility to the data is permitted for:

- the subject of the data (i.e. the patient)
- a person authorized by the subject
- a person authorized to act on behalf of the subject. This authority may not necessarily have been granted by the subject. In the case of a patient who is unable to give permission for his or her own care, a carer may be appointed by an authorized authority.
- a person with power of attorney. This will be a person authorized by the subject through legal process to deal with the subject's interests. This may occur if the subject has left the country for an extended period or has moved permanently and requires their ocular health record to be provided through an appointee granted power of attorney.

If a patient, or someone authorized by or on behalf of the patient, wants access to the personal or sensitive personal data, this request has to be made, in writing, to the practitioner (s7(1) Data Protection Act 1998). The practitioner has 40 calendar days to respond to the request. If response is not made within the specified time and further requests for data are ignored, the person applying for the data can complain to the Information Commissioner or, if they wish to seek compensation, pursue the matter through the courts. Although taking such a matter to court is not common, the practitioner should not neglect requests for data that are made under the Data Protection Act 1998. It must always be remembered that a patient can also make a complaint about a practitioner to the professional or disciplinary body. This body may not have the authority to order compliance with legislation but it does have the power to reprimand a practitioner who is seen to ignore reasonable requests from a patient.

What types of 'data' are protected?

Not all data are protected or can be accessed under the Data Protection Act 1998. The definition of what types of 'data' are protected does not depend just on the nature of the data but also on how they are recorded, stored and processed. The Data Protection Act 1998 is concerned with data that are processed using equipment that works 'automatically in response to instructions given for that purpose' (s1(1)(a)), recorded in such a way that they will be processed by such equipment (s1(1)(b)), are in a 'relevant filing system' (s1(1)(c)) or are part of an 'accessible record' (s1(1)(d)).

This means that all personal data held on a computer or any other instrument are protected under the Data Protection Act 1998, and any practitioner who keeps patient records electronically must notify and register with the Information Commissioner's Office (s17(1)). Failure to notify constitutes a criminal offence (s21).

When notifying and registering, the Data Protection Act 1998 (s16) requires practitioners to supply:

- a description of the personal details that they hold
- an outline of the reasons for which data are to be used
- data sources (major sources of data will come from patients and referrals)
- to whom data may be disclosed
- any countries outside the European Economic Area to which data may be directly or indirectly transferred.

Manual data

If records are on paper (i.e. held manually), there is no need to register with the Information Commissioner's Office (s17(2) Data Protection Act 1998). Since the Data Protection Act 1998 became law, there has been some uncertainty regarding data held manually and whether or not manual data constitute 'data' as defined by the Act. In order to fall under the definition of the 'data', manual data have to be 'organised in a relevant filing system', but the very definition of a 'relevant filing system' is vague. The Data Protection Act (s1(1)) defines a relevant filing system as:

> "... structured either by reference to the individual or to criteria relating to individuals, in such a way that specific information relating to a particular individual is readily accessible."

The lack of clarity in the definition was addressed in a recent court case (Michael John Durant v Financial Services Authority [2003]) and the judgment given provided some assistance with what can be treated as a 'relevant filing system'. It was described as one that is 'so structured and/or indexed as to enable easy location within it or any subfiles of specific information about the data subject that he has requested'. What this means is that the information needs to be filed in such a way that data can be readily acquired. From this it could be inferred that a really messy filing system or one that has a complex coding would not be a 'relevant filing system', nor would it be 'accessible'. An easier means of deciding what manual data fall under the definition of the Data Protection Act 1998 is to apply a simple test suggested by the Information Commissioner's Office. This *temp test* suggests that if a temporary employee, who was completely unfamiliar with the nature of the work done in the practice, was able easily to extract specific data about a patient, then the system would be 'accessible' and classed as a 'relevant filing system'.

If manual data are within a relevant filing system or part of an accessible record, such data will be covered under the Data Protection Act 1998. This means that, even though there would be no need to register with the Information Commissioner's Office, compliance with the eight data protection principles is still required.

When disclosure must be made

There are a number of reasons, prescribed by law, that require a practitioner to breach confidentiality of the patient and disclose personal or sensitive personal data. It is worth noting that healthcare practitioners cannot protect the confidentiality of their patients to the extent that can be invoked by legal practitioners with respect to their clients. If legal practitioners are put into a position where they need to divulge confidential information given by a client in order to uphold the law, they can claim 'professional compromise' and withdraw from the case without disclosing any confidential information. The same privilege is not extended to healthcare practitioners. If ordered by law to breach confidentiality and to disclose personal or sensitive personal data, healthcare practitioners are obliged to do so. The major reasons that would require disclosure are if it is:

- in the interests of national security (s28 Data Protection Act 1998)
- for public protection and safety (s31 Data Protection Act 1998)
- required to be disclosed by a court of law or in connection with legal proceedings (s35 Data Protection Act 1998)
- required by law (s172(2)(b) Road Traffic Act 1988).

The Road Traffic Act 1988 puts a duty on any person to tell police, on request, the name and address of a driver of a vehicle who may have been injured and is alleged to be guilty of an offence under the Road Traffic Act 1988.

Clinical case study

A regular patient comes in to collect his prescription. It is dispensed, he pays for it and he is given a receipt with the practice address and practitioner details on it. Shortly after, a police officer appears at the practice with the receipt in her hand. She asks whether the receipt was issued at the practice and explains that she has come to make enquiries in connection with a serious road accident that has caused a fatality. The driver who is believed to be at fault is too seriously injured to answer any questions and there was no identification of any sort found in the car. The car itself is so damaged that the numberplate is illegible. The receipt, in the driver's spectacle case, is the only piece of evidence that may help identify the driver at this stage. The police officer asks for the name and address of the patient. *In this situation the practitioner is obliged by law to give the details requested by the police officer, but nothing more. The ocular health record of the patient and any other examination details do not form part of the request. Providing these would be a breach of confidentiality.*

A practitioner can disclose personal data pertaining to a patient if the practitioner has been threatened or assaulted by the patient. Any assault or verbal abuse (if deemed to be threatening) is a criminal offence. Practitioners are entitled to be treated with respect and protected from assaults and threats. If such an incident has occurred, the police should be furnished with the name and cont.act details of the patient, but sensitive personal data, which are not relevant to the incident and are not requested, should not be disclosed.

Sharing of data, referrals, reporting

In healthcare practice, referrals need to be made and sharing of patient information between practitioners is common, and indeed essential. Shared care could not operate without regular information transfer. Communication between optometrists, ophthalmologists, general practitioners and other health professionals necessitates the sharing of personal and sensitive personal data. If practitioners work in the same practice, then they will have shared access to patient data and this is acceptable. If a referral is made, the patient should know to whom they are being referred and why. If they accept the referral, they implicitly accept that details about their health will be revealed to the practitioner to whom the referral is being made.

If a patient has an adverse reaction or a suspected adverse reaction to a medication or device, the practitioner should report this to the Medicines and Healthcare products Regulatory Agency (MHRA 2007) via the Yellow Card Scheme. Reporting the reaction requires disclosure of patient data. In such instances, the practitioner does not have to ask the consent of the patient and this is not treated as a breach of confidentiality. In practice, however, it is both courteous and respectful to inform a patient who has had an adverse or suspected adverse reaction that a report will be made. This is in the interest of the patient as well as, potentially, for the benefit and safety of other patients who may be taking a similar medication or using a similar device. The MHRA assures that confidentiality of patients is guarded.

Permitted disclosure

Disclosure is permitted to the parents, guardians and carers of patients who are not considered to be autonomous adults: children under the age of 16 years, frail or disabled patients. This is not a breach of confidentiality, although disclosure is not always mandatory. If, for example, an elderly patient wishes to share something very private with a practitioner and requests that this not be revealed to the carer, if the information is not relevant to the care of the patient the wish should be respected. Children under the age of 16 years are generally considered to be under the care of their parents and so it is not a breach of the confidentiality of the child to inform the parents about the state of the child's ocular health. Parents have a right to know this. The exception to this is a child who, although under 16 years of age, is sufficiently mature to be considered, by the practitioner, to be Gillick competent (as described in Chapter 5), i.e. able to understand the nature and consequences of the treatment and able to consent to it. Once a practitioner deems a patient to be Gillick competent, the patient should be treated as an autonomous adult and their confidentiality respected accordingly.

Children over the age of 16 years have the same right to confidentiality as autonomous adults. This means that the outcome of an examination of any patient aged 16 years or over cannot be disclosed to the parents unless the explicit permission of the patient has been sought and given.

Unintended disclosure

Whilst it is obvious that a practitioner would not wilfully or recklessly divulge personal or sensitive personal data, this can sometimes be done unintentionally. The mere act of recognizing a patient outside the practice setting and pointing out to a third party that this is a patient at the practice is a breach of confidentiality. It tells the third party that the individual has come in for an eye examination and that may lead to an inference about their state of health. The individual may not wish to have this information revealed.

Another instance in which confidentiality may be inadvertently breached can occur when the practitioner has a number of family members as patients and is asked by one family member about the ocular health or prescription of another.

The married couple

Clinical case study

A couple come into your practice and you notice that they are holding hands and are very close and attentive to each another. They are both patients at your practice and come in for routine examinations as both

Continued

have a prescription but no ocular pathology or systemic conditions that may affect vision or health of the eye. You examine the wife first and, when her consultation is finished, you invite the husband into the consulting room. On examination you find that his prescription has altered slightly, but sufficiently for him to prefer the new prescription. Whilst you are making a note of this on the record card, he casually asks whether there has been any change in the prescription of his wife.

Should you tell him?

The answer to the above question is 'no'. Although this is a very close couple that could be expected to share far more intimate information with one another than the magnitude of a spectacle prescription, the information they share is communicated directly between the pair. It does not mean that a third party, such as a healthcare practitioner, should assume the liberty of conveying such information about one spouse to the other. Both husband and wife are patients, and the relationship that each has with the practitioner should be treated as two separate practitioner–patient relationships. A prescription is sensitive personal information, and the husband should not be told anything about the results of his wife's examination without her consent. In practice, where the practitioner and patients know one another well, the consequence of such disclosure may not lead to any complaint or ramifications, but the confidentiality of each patient should always be maintained.

The unmarried father

Parents are always given the details of their children's health and the outcome measures of any examination, because the parent is deemed to be responsible for the child and therefore has a right to know. An exception to parental right to know applies to the unmarried father. If parents are not married, the father does not share the same rights as the mother. A recent exception has been introduced: if the child was born after 1 December 2003 and the father was present at the registration of birth, he has parental responsibility and is thus permitted access to the same information as the married father (s111(2) Adoption and Children Act 2002). In any other case, he must be granted parental responsibility (which can be obtained through a court) before any disclosure about any aspect of the health of the child can be made to him. If there is any doubt about the marital status of the parents of a child patient, and the father of the patient requests clinical or treatment details about the child, the practitioner ought to enquire about parental responsibility before disclosing any information.

SUMMARY

Confidential information that is found in the patient database of every practice has some protection in law. Respect for confidentiality is also an ethical obligation. There will be instances in which exceptions to protecting personal data need to be made and where the law offers limited guidance. The decision about whether or not to disclose information in such cases rests with the practitioner; whatever decision is made, it should always be properly justified.

References

Adoption and Children Act 2002 Office of Public Sector Information. Online. Available: http://www.opsi.gov.uk/acts/acts2002/20020038.htm

College of Optometrists 2007 Code of ethics and guidelines for professional conduct: 26. Examining children and vulnerable adults. Online. Available: http://www.college-optometrists.org/index.aspx/pcms/site.publication.Ethics_Guidelines.Ethics_Guidelines_home/

Data Protection Act 1998 Office of Public Sector Information. Online. Available: http://www.opsi.gov.uk/acts/acts1998/19980029.htm

Department of Health 2003 The Victoria Climbié inquiry. Report of an inquiry by Lord Laming. The Stationery Office, London. Online. Available: http://www.dh.gov.uk/en/Publicationsandstatistics/Publications/PublicationsPolicyAndGuidance/DH_4008654

Medicines and Healthcare products Regulatory Agency 2007 Reporting suspected adverse drug reactions. Online. Available: http://www.mhra.gov.uk/home/idcplg?IdcService=SS_GET_PAGE&nodeId=287

Michael John Durant v Financial Services Authority [2003] EWCA Civ 1746, Court of Appeal (Civil Division)

Road Traffic Act 1988 Office of Public Sector Information. Online. Available: http://www.opsi.gov.uk/acts/acts1988/Ukpga_19880052_en_1.htm

8

Collegiality and employment law

COLLEGIALITY

The ethical principles described in preceding chapters are concerned primarily with the patient–practitioner relationship. In healthcare practice, as in any other employment, the behaviour towards and relationship between practitioners is also vitally important. It underpins the way in which a practice is run, it can affect the way that patients are treated (an unhappy or disgruntled practitioner is unlikely to put his or her best effort into patient care), and it can impact on the profession and its reputation.

Any relationship involves giving and receiving. In the patient–practitioner relationship there is a one-sided provision of help and care: the patient seeks help and care, the practitioner has the training, skills and knowledge to provide that care. The ethical principles that guide this relationship reflect the different roles of the patient and practitioner, and remind the latter that he or she is primarily responsible for fostering the relationship.

A relationship between colleagues is generally considered to be one in which both parties are, more or less, on a par in terms of giving and receiving. If two colleagues are indeed of equal rank, it is reasonable to expect that responsibility for maintaining the relationship should be shared. However, the notion that all work-based relationships are between individuals of similar status in the workplace is not always correct. It very much depends on the stringency in the definition of 'colleague'. If the term colleague is used to define individuals who work together in positions of equal grading, parity in the relationship may be assumed. Yet, the common use of the term 'colleague' can be broader than this and there is often a difference in seniority, responsibility and experience between employees who regard one another as colleagues. The senior optometrist who owns the practice and the junior optometrist who has just passed pre-registration exams and works in the practice are colleagues, yet a number of factors that can impact on the relationship distinguish one from the other. The senior optometrist may be the employer as well as the mentor of the junior colleague. The two will have different roles in the relationship and each will have certain expectations of the other. These expectations should always be reasonable. The senior optometrist will be responsible for sharing and imparting knowledge and experience in clinical skills, practice management and dealing with patients. He or she can reasonably expect the newly qualified practitioner to be enthusiastic and willing to learn from the mentor. The younger optometrist can expect to be taught and to learn from mistakes made and, at times, from constructive suggestions for improvement. His or her responsibility will grow with time as the skills necessary to cope with it are learned. The younger colleague can expect to learn from and be guided by the senior colleague and mentor.

Whatever definition of collegiality is used, the essential components of this ethical principle are mutual respect and understanding for the other person and for their role in the healthcare team. The behaviour with respect to others should extend beyond the boundaries of a single profession. The optometrist and the ophthalmologist, to whom patients are referred, can consider themselves to be colleagues in the broader context of eye care. Indeed, the characteristics of collegiality should be integral in all relationships between individuals who work together in healthcare practice. The emphasis of collegiality is becoming more important as the concept of team working and shared care develops. Respect and understanding between practitioners and non-practitioners in the workplace promotes good working relationships and shared care is ultimately for the benefit of the patient.

It is relatively easy to be collegiate towards and understanding of a colleague with whom we get along. Yet, there will always be people with whom we have little, if anything, in common, and those who have different opinions, attitudes, perspectives and behaviour. When a person is judged on the basis of these differences and treated in an unfair or discriminatory manner as a result, collegiality has been replaced with prejudice.

Generalizations and prejudice

The avoidance of prejudice requires an awareness and admission that it exists and an active attempt to deal with it and ultimately to eradicate it.

Ethical principles can be considered as generalizations because they are applied, in clinical practice, in a way that is not selective. For example, a practitioner does not apply beneficence to patients over a certain age and non-maleficence to those who are younger. In many aspects of life, people generalize because this helps in organizing thoughts and ideas, in dealing with certain matters and in planning for future eventualities. Society uses generalizations when it classes people in certain categories, allowing some people greater rights than others. The age of 18 years as the age at which people are allowed to vote is an example of this. Generalization brings order and organization into life and, if applied properly, can be effective. When generalizations are used in the wrong way they can lead to prejudice. This can happen when generalization is applied to categorize people, as this leads to pre-judging a person on the basis of the category to which they are considered to belong (Allport 1954, cited by Plous 2003). It may be an instinctive response: a bad experience during a first visit to a foreign country can lead to prejudice formed about all of its citizens without rationalizing that in every national group there will be those who are helpful and friendly and those who are not.

In law, the defendant cannot be pre-judged before a trial. Outside the formal legal system, opinion about another should be considered in the same way, for if prejudice is left unchecked it can become integrated with stereotypical and unreasonable beliefs and start to be treated as reasonable. The individual against whom prejudice is levelled has not been given a 'fair trial'. It is easy to fall into this cycle of pre-judging a group of people, endowing them with certain characteristics and traits (usually based on the experiences of one or a small number of the perceived group), and then forming an immediate opinion of anyone else who is considered to belong to that group.

It may be seen as entirely unreasonable to most people to label all football supporters as hooligans on the basis that some people behave inappropriately at football matches. In a similar way, it is highly unlikely that any reasoning individual will treat all teenagers as a menace to society because a minority may terrorize their neighbourhood. There may be more people, however, willing to judge all teenagers within a particularly rough neighbourhood as troublemakers. Any well behaved young person living in the vicinity, or maybe even passing through, is at risk of being unfairly labelled and potentially treated prejudicially.

Efforts to restrict prejudice in society have manifested largely in the form of rules and legislative means to prohibit discrimination. This has been effective in raising awareness and preventing actions that result in injustice on the basis of prejudice. Outlawing actions, however, cannot guarantee a change in outlook and mindset. A person who feels prejudice towards those of another race will not express these feeling openly as the law does not allow racial discrimination. Such a person sitting on a selection committee interviewing candidates for a job may, however, find covert ways of eliminating an applicant because he or she belongs to that race. Unless the prejudice is acknowledged, its roots explored and the underlying issues confronted and eliminated, prejudice will remain and will lead to discrimination and non-collegial behaviour.

Every person can, in certain situations, be prone to pre-judging another person or group of people and this can lead to the development of a prejudiced attitude. An active effort is required to desist from this. Prejudice has no place in any aspect of life; it should be especially avoided in professional practice.

Collegial relations with fellow practitioners

In healthcare practice, as in any occupation where professional people work together, there is an understanding that colleagues will support and not undermine one another. Within a practice the care of patients is shared. This means that there is a collective responsibility for patient welfare and for maintaining good patient–practitioner relations. Undermining or unfairly criticizing a colleague or their performance to a patient is not collegial and can reflect as badly or even more negatively on the critic as on the subject of the criticism. This behaviour serves no purpose and competition for patients by practitioners who work in the same practice is counterproductive.

Some form of competition does exist between practices as practitioners strive to increase or at least maintain their patient base. This, however, does not mean that practitioners have the right to solicit for patients by undermining colleagues who work in other practices. Sometimes a patient may present with a prescription with which he or she is not satisfied, obtained from another practitioner. Even if the former practitioner has erred, it is not collegial to emphasize this to the patient. Mistakes can happen and everyone is prone to err from time to time. Poor or sloppy practice is inexcusable but it does not justify making disparaging comments about a fellow practitioner.

Should support for colleagues be absolute?

Collegiality does not mean supporting colleagues under any circumstances, regardless of what they do or do not do. In every profession there will be members who make mistakes through lack of competence, misunderstanding, or inadvertently. There may even be instances in which a professional behaves in a way that undermines their status and reflects badly on the profession. Collegiality includes reminding a colleague, who is doing something that is not acceptable, that they should stop and, if necessary, asking them to rectify any harm caused by the wrong-doing. The transgression may require reporting a colleague to the appropriate person, perhaps the practice manager or a senior practitioner. A colleague could be under-performing, missing certain tests, issuing prescriptions that are not grossly erroneous but not quite correct. There could be an explanation for this: personal problems, health or family concerns. Colleagues in such a position should be given help and support, at all times remembering that patient care cannot be allowed to suffer.

More serious misdemeanours, incompetence that could harm a patient or misconduct may require reporting to the professional body. Criminal acts and activities – theft, assault, deliberate harming of a patient – should be reported to the police. Collegiality does not include covering up the misdeeds of another professional. It does include discretion. Unless requested (by the professional body, police or other appropriate authority), it is not collegial to discuss and publicize the errors another practitioner may have made or the actions that have been taken against him or her.

Recognizing problems

Even in practices and workplaces where colleagues are supportive, respectful of and friendly to one another, situations may arise where collegiality becomes threatened. This can happen when a colleague starts to behave in a way that is out of character. If this change has a negative effect on others, collegial relations may become strained. Often this can happen as a result of rumour, gossip or simple misunderstandings. There may be other reasons why a practitioner starts to alter in their attitude and behaviour to others. It is not unusual to find that sometimes the good work of one employee is perceived to be a threat by other colleagues to their own performance. This leads to resentment and eventual erosion of collegiality. Such cases occur most commonly in workplaces, companies and institutions where employees are expected to meet targets and are assessed on their output. This manner of monitoring people, although designed to help improve work performance, often has an opposite and adverse effect on collegial relationships (and may not have the desired effect on productivity), especially if employees are pitted against one another. In healthcare practice, the common goal is to help the patient. The result may not always be as readily apparent as are the measurable outcomes in other occupations and the patient may not always express gratitude to the practitioner who contributed the most to their care. It could seem as though efforts have gone unrecognized. At such times, it helps to remember that patient care is a team effort, and in a team all colleagues should be valued. Problems can also arise when a new colleague joins the team:

Case study

John, Mike and Sam are optometrists who work in the same practice. Sam is a little younger than his colleagues and is the only one who is single. He started working at the practice about 2 years ago and found John and Mike, who had been there for some years, to be very amicable and supportive. The three practitioners have become quite close friends. They go to lunch together and for a drink after work once a week. The practice is expanding and there is a need for another practitioner. Out of the pool of applicants, Sally is found to be the best qualified and she has a particular expertise that fits into the practice specializations.

When Sally starts work she is given the same welcome and encouragement that was extended to Sam. She is invited to lunch with her colleagues and she is happy to accept. After the first couple of weeks, within which Sally and her new colleagues come to know one another better, it becomes apparent that Sally has quite a lot in common with John and Mike.

Continued

She attends the same craft class as Mike's wife and her children go to the same school as John's children. Conversation topics over lunch are less inclined to be about football and the odd joke, and more frequently concern children and family activities. Sam, who is younger than the other three, finds himself left out. He starts to resent Sally and what he perceives to be her intrusive questioning and domination of conversation topics. He suggests to Mike that maybe they could stop including Sally in all of their lunches; perhaps she should be asked to join them only a couple of times a week. Mike is surprised and asks why. Sam blurts out that since a woman has joined the practice she seems to be taking over.

Is Sam being unfair to Sally or have the other practitioners been less inclusive than they should have been?

The behaviour Sam has shown may be interpreted as a manifestation of sexism: he appears to prefer all male company and to consider a female colleague unwelcome. However, there is no indication that Sam treats Sally unfairly in the workplace. The underlying cause of Sam's resentment is the fact that he does not feel able to contribute to the sort of conversations that Sally's presence has initiated. This is not surprising; it can be extremely difficult for a single person to contribute to conversations about family life and activities of children. There is also the fact that Sam has become accustomed to a situation in which he and his colleagues socialized easily and had an established commonality of interests. The inclusion of Sally has altered this camaraderie and Sam is the only one who cannot adjust to the new arrangement. Sally appears to have 'replaced' Sam within the inner collegial circle. Indeed, if the practitioners were interviewed about collegiality and asked whether they feel fairly treated, Sam is likely to indicate that any unfair treatment has been metered out to him and not to Sally. The more senior colleagues, John and Mike, are unaware about how Sam feels, and Sally, who has had no previous experience of the social interactions between her three colleagues before her arrival, could not know how her inclusion has altered collegial relations for Sam. If the situation continues, Sam is likely to become more resentful, may make his feelings about Sally known and, eventually, Sam may even leave to find another position. If he does so, he will leave a practice, where he used to enjoy working, with bitter feelings. If Sally stops being included in social events, she is likely to look at the most obvious difference between herself and her colleagues – she is female – and come to the conclusion that she is being discriminated against on the grounds of gender. Neither outcome – Sam leaving or Sally feeling that she is being discriminated against – would be pleasant and both could be averted. John and Mike could steer some of the lunchtime conversations to topics with which Sam is familiar. Sam would then stop resenting Sally and collegiality between the two would be free to develop. When colleagues work well together, common interests often emerge. Sam and Sally may find that they like the same foods or have a similar taste in music. Early recognition and resolution of a problem prevents it from escalating into a demise of collegiality, resulting in bad feelings, hurt and even actions that may lead to litigation.

How sensitive colleagues ought to be to one another is like asking how beneficent should a practitioner be towards his or her patients. It depends on the work situation, the practitioners, their relationships in and out of work, and ultimately on the individual. There are people who do not wish to combine work and social life and, whilst they may treat colleagues with respect and courtesy in the workplace, they are disinclined to maintain contact with and therefore be concerned about attitudes of colleagues outside this environment. They may argue that it should not matter how uncomfortable or excluded a colleague feels over a lunch or other out-of-work activity; such instances will sometimes occur in social interactions. As long as colleagues are treated fairly during working hours, and allowed to do their job without hindrance, this is as far as collegiality should extend. That is very much a matter of personal ethics and the situation in the working environment. If the practice is one in which all practitioners have little in common outside work and choose not to socialize, it may be applicable. However, where collegiate relations are such that socializing occurs frequently and people often lunch together or meet after work, the way in which a colleague is treated in a social setting should not be ignored or neglected. Whilst socializing should try to be inclusive, there should never be any expectation on a colleague to join in and attend if they are reluctant to do so. Not all people find social settings with colleagues and fellow employees pleasant, and some can even feel ill at ease at functions and parties organized for special occasions. A colleague who does not wish to socialize outside work should not be labelled, considered odd or treated less favourably during working hours than other colleagues. Differences and choices should be respected.

Unwelcome intervention

Collegiality may sometimes be tested and attempts at help refused. A colleague may become withdrawn and distant. Questions about what may be wrong are met with an unexpected rebuff that could easily be interpreted as rudeness. When people work together closely and get on well with one another there may be a presumption that problems that may occur in other aspects of life can be shared. This presumption will not always be correct. Some problems are difficult to share and others may not be considered appropriate to divulge to colleagues. In addition, what is deemed appropriate or not will vary from individual to individual. Attempts to find out what is wrong, when a colleague is reluctant to say what may be troubling them, could be interpreted as intrusive. Respecting the privacy of others and their right to protect what they would rather not disclose should always be respected, even when it appears unusual or when others think it would be in a colleague's better interest to share their problems.

Case study

An academic was suffering from anorexia nervosa and was in denial about the condition. Concerned colleagues reported her to the head of department, asking for action to be taken to help her. The head of department referred the matter to the head of personnel, who felt that he had no authority to take action. Her work performance was not suffering, although as time went on she was ever more frequently ill. Further attempts at intervention by colleagues were seen as intrusive and unwelcome, and after some time the academic died from internal organ failure.

This case is based on an occurrence at an Australian University.

EMPLOYMENT LAW

"At its best employment law is logical, dynamic, interesting and real. At its worst it resembles the M25."

(Holland & Burnett 2003)

Unless a person is genuinely self-employed, that is, they have not entered into any contract of employment, service or apprenticeship, then they are an employee and the work they do is regulated and covered by employment law (The Employment Rights Act 1996, sections 230(1) and 230(2)). This includes the laws made in the United Kingdom and those that are incorporated from European law. Employment law protects employees and employers from unfair practice and wrongful behaviour in the workplace. This protection is needed because the employer–employee relationship is not a relationship of equals: the employee depends on the employer for a job. The employee works under the instruction or supervision of the employer and if the employer brings an end to the employment the employee is left without a job. For this reason, there needs to be a contract of employment signed by both employer and employee that incorporates terms guaranteeing the employee some security and rights. Without a contract and the protection of the law, the employer–employee relationship would be akin to that of master and servant. (Although the term 'servant', a term that predates 'employee', is still used in certain areas of employment, for instance when referring to civil servants employed in government departments, there ought not to be any aspect of servitude involved.)

Employment law may appear at times to be chaotic and even bizarre. This may be because the cases that make headlines in the press are often those that highlight extreme situations: sexual discrimination in professions that have been traditionally male bastions or blatant racial discrimination. It may also be because employment law is an area of law that develops at a faster rate than other areas and hence changes and new developments are more frequent. The aspects that impact strongly on employment issues, such as avoidance of discrimination, fair treatment of employees and human rights, are developing areas that are influenced by European law, itself a rapidly evolving area. Changes to employment law can also be made in response to political and/or economic factors.

Legislation that protects against discrimination on specific grounds

There are a number of legislative provisions that prohibit discrimination in the workplace on the grounds of race, gender and disability, and, more recently, regulations that protect employees from discrimination on religious grounds, age and part-time work have been introduced. The Acts described apply to England, Scotland and Wales, and similar provisions have been made for Northern Ireland.

It is important to remember that the law is concerned with actions and how actions affect people. It is not concerned with opinions. Legislation against discrimination on any ground outlaws only the actions; it does not prohibit prejudice. This ought to be dealt with by the individual who holds such opinions.

Gender-based discrimination

The Sex Discrimination Act 1975, which applies to England, Scotland and Wales, outlaws discrimination on the grounds of gender, marital status or being in a civil partnership. It is also unlawful to discriminate against an employee who has undergone gender reassignment. The Sex Discrimination (Northern Ireland) Order 1976 makes similar provisions in Northern Ireland.

The legislation describes different types of gender-based discrimination:

- *Direct* – treating an employee less favourably than other employees in the same circumstances on the grounds of his or her gender or because he or she is married. Telling a female practitioner that as part of her job she is expected to make tea and coffee for and clean up after male colleagues would be an example of direct discrimination.
- *Indirect* – requiring employees to comply with conditions or practices that would lead to an employee being disadvantaged because of his or her gender or because he or she is married. In a particular practice, a piece of reasonably heavy equipment sometimes needs to be moved from one consulting room to another. To introduce a requirement that the practitioner who needs the equipment is responsible for moving it may cause difficulties for a female practitioner, who lacks the strength of her male colleagues. This may amount to indirect discrimination.
- *Victimization* – treating an employee less favourably than other employees because the employee has made or intends to make a complaint on the grounds of gender-based inequality. Victimization claims can also be made by ex-employees who had made a complaint against the employer whilst still in employment (Sex Discrimination Act 1975 (Amendment) Regulations

2003). Failing to provide a reference for an ex-employee who has made an allegation of sexual discrimination could constitute victimization.

- *Harassment/sexual harassment* – intimidating, being hostile towards or humiliating an employee on the grounds of gender; actions or comments that are lewd or suggestive; unwelcome sexual attention; or creating an environment that another employee finds offensive or degrading. This form of discrimination also covers treatment of an employee after the employee has rejected or submitted to unwanted conduct, if that treatment is less favourable than it would have been had the employee not rejected or submitted to that conduct.

Racial discrimination

The Race Relations Act 1976, which applies to England, Scotland and Wales, prohibits discrimination on the grounds of 'colour, nationality, race, ethnic or national origin'. Similar legislative provisions have been made for Northern Ireland in the Race Relations (Northern Ireland) Order 1997.

This covers all forms of employment including partnerships, but in the latter case there is a small provision for partnerships with small firms. For firms with six or more partners it is unlawful to prevent someone from becoming partner on all grounds cited in the act ('colour, nationality, race, ethnic or national origin'). For firms with fewer than six partners, the prohibition applies only to discrimination on the grounds of 'race, ethnic or national origin'.

The different types of racial discrimination defined by law are similar to those described for sex discrimination:

- *Direct* – treating an employee less favourably, on racial grounds, than other employees in the same circumstances. An example of this is paying the only practitioner who comes from a non-British background a lower salary than the other practitioners even though all work the same number of hours and see similar numbers of patients.
- *Indirect* – imposing conditions or policies that appear to be fair because they apply to all employees, but which are difficult to meet or detrimental for members of a particular racial group. Insisting that all practitioners have their heads uncovered whilst in the practice is indirect discrimination against members of racial groups (Jews, Sikhs) for whom practice requires

that a head covering is worn. The Race Relations Act 1976 deals only with indirect discrimination on the basis of colour and nationality. The Race Relations Act 1976 (Amendment) Regulations 2003 and the Race Relations Order (Amendment) Regulations (Northern Ireland) 2003 have extended indirect discrimination to cover grounds of race, ethnic or national origin. A requirement that all personal calls, including those made in the tea-room at lunchtime, have to be made in English may appear to be non-discriminatory. However, such a rule would make it difficult for a practitioner, whose national origin is not English, and who needs to check on her young child by speaking to her baby sitter in their native tongue.

- *Victimization* – treating an employee less favourably than other employees in the same circumstances because the employee has made or intends to make a complaint of racial discrimination. Victimization claims can be made by ex-employees who had made a complaint for racial discrimination against the employer whilst still in employment (Race Relations Act 1976 (Amendment) Regulations 2003).
- *Harassment* – intimidating, offending or humiliating an employee on grounds of race, ethnic or nation origin. This is prohibited by the Race Relations Act 1976 (Amendment) Regulations 2003 and the Race Relations Order (Amendment) Regulations (Northern Ireland) 2003. Imitating, in a nasty way, the accent of a practitioner whose first language is not English could amount to a charge of harassment. If an employee is harassed on the grounds of colour or nationality, this could be treated as direct discrimination.

Is racial discrimination in healthcare practice ever allowed?

There are exceptions to the Race Relations Act but these should not be treated as occasions in which discrimination on the grounds of race is permitted. Rather, they are situations in which there is good reason or a need specifically to employ someone from a particular race. The exceptions that apply to healthcare practice concern situations in which race, ethnicity or national origin are genuine occupational requirements or where belonging to a particular racial group is a genuine occupational qualification (Race Relations Act 1976 (Amendment) Regulations 2003, Race Relations Order (Amendment) Regulations (Northern Ireland) 2003).

An example where this may be implemented is in a health centre that deals exclusively with patients who do not speak English.

It would not be treated as discriminatory if the health centre sought to employ a practitioner who spoke the same language as the patients. In this case, the post requires the added qualification of a foreign language. If this language is not taught in schools but spoken only by those who belong to a particular racial or ethnic group, the health centre would be justified in employing a practitioner who is a member of that group.

Discrimination on the basis of religion or faith

Although the Race Relations Act does not cover discrimination on the basis of religion or belief, some religious groups (Jews, Sikhs) are also recognized as racial groups. The Race Relations Act also covers discrimination against a religious group if this is indirect racial discrimination (e.g. discrimination against a Muslim employee that is veiled attempt at discrimination because the person is from a Pakistani background).

The Employment Equality (Religion or Belief) Regulations 2003 strengthen the law against religious discrimination, outlawing direct and indirect forms of discrimination and harassment on the grounds of religion or belief as well as protecting against victimization of an individual who has made a complaint about being the victim of discrimination on religious or faith-based grounds. More serious offences of stirring up hatred against an individual because of his or her religion or indeed because the individual does not have a religious belief are prohibited under the Racial and Religious Hatred Act 2006, which is applied to England and Wales only. In Northern Ireland discrimination on the grounds of religious belief is prohibited by the Fair Employment (Northern Ireland) Act 1989 and the Fair Employment and Treatment (Northern Ireland) Order 1998.

Discrimination on the grounds of disability

One of the most significant changes made to employment law in recent times has been the impact of the Disability Discrimination Act 1995. The Disability Discrimination Act 1995 has been discussed in relation to how it is applied to patients in the chapter on Justice. This Act also deals with preventing discrimination in the workplace. It is against the law for an employer to discriminate against a disabled applicant in deciding about which applicant should get the post, the terms on which the post is offered, or refusing the job to the disabled applicant on the basis of the disability.

Case study

A position for a part-time optometrist is advertised. Among the applicants is a person with a disability. She had a previous injury to her back and, although she is able to conduct all examinations on patients, she can work for only half a day at a time. The advert for the job states that 'an optometrist is needed for three half-days a week, times to be negotiated'. The applicant has skills and qualifications that are better than all other applicants, but the post is not offered to her and she is told that this is because a practitioner is needed for at least one full day per week.

The terms of the job have been altered so that the disabled applicant could not fulfil the requirements. This is unlawful under section 4(1)(b) of the Disability Discrimination Act 1995.

An employer cannot treat a disabled employee less favourably than other employees or dismiss a disabled employee because of the disability. The disabled employee must be provided with the same opportunities for promotion, training, transfer or any other benefits that are offered to other employees in the same employment.

As for disabled patients (discussed in Chapter 6 on Justice), there is a duty on the employer to make reasonable adjustments to the workplace and practices so that the disabled employee is not at a 'substantial disadvantage' compared with other employees. The list of possible steps that may need to be taken includes making adjustments to premises, modifying procedures for testing, making an interpreter available, arranging for training and providing supervision.

When the Disability Discrimination Act 1995 came into force there was an exemption for small businesses limited to employing fewer than 20 people. This was subsequently amended to apply to workplaces with fewer than 15 people before the exemption was removed entirely (Disability Discrimination Act 1995 (Amendment) Regulations 2003).

Discrimination on the basis of age or sexual orientation, part-time and fixed-term employment

More recently, protection against discrimination has been extended to cover grounds of sexual orientation (Employment Equality (Sexual Orientation) Regulations 2003, Employment Equality (Sexual Orientation) Regulations (Northern Ireland) 2003). This includes discrimination based on perceived or actual sexual orientation as well on the basis of association.

Since 1 October 2006 it has been illegal to discriminate against an employee on the grounds of age (Employment Equality (Age) Regulations 2006, Employment Equality (Age) Regulations (Northern Ireland) 2006). As with other grounds, legislation prohibiting discrimination on the grounds of age or sexual orientation covers direct and indirect discrimination, victimization and harassment.

Employees who work part-time hours or are on fixed-term contracts have their rights to be treated as fairly as their full-time colleagues in permanent posts protected under the Part-time Workers (Prevention of Less Favourable Treatment) Regulations 2000 and the Fixed-Term Employees (Prevention of Less Favourable Treatment) Regulations 2002, respectively. Comparable regulations apply in Northern Ireland.

Is positive discrimination permitted?

In situations where there is an under-representation of certain groups, policies given the label of 'positive discrimination' are introduced. This is a poor use of terminology because in practice any form of discrimination is outlawed. To discriminate positively for one group of people will inevitably lead to an unfavourable discrimination against another group. Whilst encouraging members of under-represented groups to apply, openly favouring applicants from these groups over other applicants is not allowed.

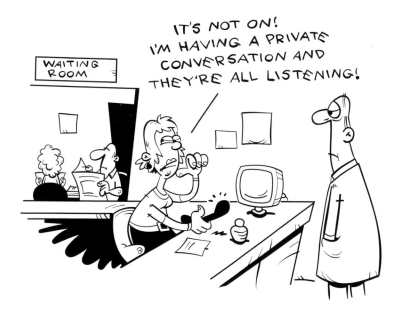

Bullying at work

Unfortunately, bullying does occur in the workplace and there is no specific piece of legislation that is concerned with bullying *per se*. However, there are laws that take into account the effect of bullying on employees. The Health and Safety at Work etc. Act 1974 places the onus on an employer to ensure that employees are protected from any behaviour that may by detrimental to their physical or mental/psychological well-being. Under the Employment Rights Act 1996, an employee is protected from suffering from detriment at work. Until recently, making a claim for bullying at work was complicated by the lack of specific legislation prohibiting bullying and the fact that any claim against another employee, if taken to an external court or employment tribunal, necessitated a claim against the employer and not the bullying employee. A recent court case, which permitted the Protection from Harassment Act 1997 to be used in an employment situation, has altered this.

The Protection from Harassment Act 1997 was intended to protect against harassment by individuals and to prohibit stalking. It was thought not to apply in employment law cases where claims are made against an employer and not against the individual responsible for the bullying and harassment. A landmark judgment in the case of Majrowski v Guy's and St Thomas' NHS Trust [2005] [2006] set a precedent and sent a stark warning to employers that they could now be vicariously liable for actions of an employee who bullies or harasses another employee during the course of employment. The bully would no longer be able to 'hide' behind the employer because, under the Protection from Harassment Act 1997, the bully is the prime perpetrator. Furthermore, an action taken under the Act gives a much longer limitation period than one taken through the usual route of internal procedures and employment tribunal; the Act allows victims of bullying and harassment up to 6 years to make a claim.

Majrowski v Guy's and St Thomas' NHS Trust [2005] [2006]

William Majrowski, who worked for Guy's and St Thomas' NHS Trust, made a complaint about bullying and harassment by his line manager. In the county court, a claim under the Protection from Harassment Act 1997 was brought against the Trust. The single judge in the county court rejected the claim on the grounds that the Protection from Harassment Act could be used only to protect against harassment and bullying by individuals and so the employer could not be held liable. Majrowski appealed against this judgment and the Court of Appeal (in a two to one judgment) found in Majrowski's favour: that an employer could be held vicariously liable, under the Protection from Harassment Act 1997, for the actions of an employee towards another employee. The Trust appealed this decision and the matter went to the House of Lords, where the Law Lords agreed unanimously with the Court of Appeal decision.

Bullying is an indication of immaturity and fear. Mature, intelligent and accomplished individuals who are secure in their own abilities do not bully others. The bully in the workplace is often an employee who has an over-inflated opinion of self and tends to target another employee who is good at his or her job because the bully perceives this as a threat. If a bully rises to a position of power, the workplace environment can become very damaging. It will be damaging for the victim(s) of the bullying as well as for those employees who stand back and may even support the bully. These are likely to be employees who lack skills and abilities to reach the positions they covet and so rally around the bully in the hope that he or she will reward their support with, what are effectively, undeserved promotions. Too frequently this happens in large organizations, but it can happen in workplaces with a relatively small number of employees. Victimization of competent employees and promotion of the less competent can only lead to an unhealthy work environment and the inevitable fall in productivity and standards. All employees who have any integrity, practise ethically and treat colleagues with respect should act to counter bullying wherever it occurs.

SUMMARY

Collegiality is an ethical principle that relates to relationships between practitioners. It requires respecting colleagues and individual differences, whilst maintaining requisite practice standards and working together for the benefit of the patient. Care should be taken to avoid any form of prejudice and unfair judgement of others. The law offers protection against workplace discrimination, on the grounds of gender, race, disability, age, religion and sexual orientation, as well as protecting employees who work part-time or are on fixed-term contracts.

References

Allport G 1954 The nature of prejudice. Cited by Plous S 2003 The psychology of prejudice, stereotyping, and discrimination: an overview. In: Plous S (ed.) Understanding prejudice and discrimination. McGraw-Hill, New York, pp 3–48

Disability Discrimination Act 1995 Online. Available: http://www.opsi.gov.uk/acts/acts1995/Ukpga_19950050_en_1.htm

Disability Discrimination Act 1995 (Amendment) Regulations 2003 Online. Available: http://www.opsi.gov.uk/si/si2003/20031673.htm#7

Employment Act 1989 Online. Available: http://www.opsi.gov.uk/acts/acts1989/Ukpga_19890038_en_1.htm

Employment Equality (Age) Regulations 2006 Online. Available: http://www.opsi.gov.uk/si/si2006/20061031.htm#3

Employment Equality (Age) Regulations (Northern Ireland) 2006 Online. Available: http://www.opsi.gov.uk/Sr/sr2006/20060261.htm

Employment Equality (Religion or Belief) Regulations 2003 Online. Available: http://www.opsi.gov.uk/si/si2003/20031660.htm#3

Employment Equality (Sexual Orientation) Regulations 2003. Online. Available: http://www.opsi.gov.uk/SI/si2003/20031661.htm

Employment Equality (Sexual Orientation) Regulations (Northern Ireland) 2003 Online. Available: http://www.opsi.gov.uk/sr/sr2003/20030497.htm

Employment Rights Act 1996 Online. Available: http://www.opsi.gov.uk/acts/acts1996/1996018.htm

Fair Employment (Northern Ireland) Act 1989 Online. Available: http://www.opsi.gov.uk/ACTS/acts1989/Ukpga_19890032_en_1.htm

Fair Employment and Treatment (Northern Ireland) Order 1998 Online. Available: http://www.opsi.gov.uk/si/si1998/19983162.htm

Fixed-term Employees (Prevention of Less Favourable Treatment) Regulations 2002 Online. Available: http://www.opsi.gov.uk/si/si2002/20022034.htm

Fixed-term Employees (Prevention of Less Favourable Treatment) Regulations (Northern Ireland) 2002 Online. Available: http://www.opsi.gov.uk/sr/sr2002/nisr_20020298_en.pdf

Health and Safety at Work etc. Act 1974 The UK Statute Law Database, Ministry of Justice. Online. Available: http://www.statutelaw.gov.uk/

Holland J, Burnett S 2003 LPC employment law (Blackstone Legal Practice Course Guide). Oxford University Press, Oxford

Majrowski v Guy's and St Thomas' NHS Trust [2005] 2 WLR 1503, [2005] EWCA Civ 251, [2006] UKHL 34. Online. Available: http://www.bailii.org/

Part-time Workers (Prevention of Less Favourable Treatment) Regulations 2000 Online. Available: http://www.opsi.gov.uk/si/si2000/20001551.htm#5

Part-time Workers (Prevention of Less Favourable Treatment) Regulations (Northern Ireland) 2000 Online. Available: http://www.opsi.gov.uk/sr/sr2000/nisr_20000219_en.pdf

Protection from Harassment Act 1997 Online. Available: http://www.opsi.gov.uk/acts/acts1997/1997040.htm

Race Relations Act 1976 The UK Statute Law Database, Ministry of Justice. Online. Available: http://www.statutelaw.gov.uk/

Race Relations Act 1976 (Amendment) Regulations 2003 Online. Available: http://www.opsi.gov.uk/SI/si2003/20031626.htm

Race Relations (Northern Ireland) Order 1997 Online. Available: http://www.opsi.gov.uk/si/si1997/70869—a.htm#3

Race Relations Order (Amendment) Regulations (Northern Ireland) 2003 Online. Available: http://www.opsi.gov.uk/Sr/sr2003/20030341.htm

Racial and Religious Hatred Act 2006 Online. Available: http://www.opsi.gov.uk/acts/acts2006/20060001.htm

Sex Discrimination Act 1975 The UK Statute Law Database, Ministry of Justice. Online. Available: http://www.statutelaw.gov.uk/

Sex Discrimination Act 1975 (Amendment) Regulations 2003 Online. Available: http://www.opsi.gov.uk/si/si2003/20031657.htm

Sex Discrimination (Northern Ireland) Order 1976 The UK Statute Law Database, Ministry of Justice. Online. Available: http://www.statutelaw.gov.uk/

9

The tort of negligence

"The rule that you are to love your neighbour becomes in law: You must not injure your neighbour."

Lord Atkin (ruling on Donoghue v Stevenson [1932])

One of the most feared incidents in the career of a practitioner is a charge of negligence alleged by a patient. Legal actions, particularly in cases citing professional wrongdoing, are at best unpleasant and at worst can be extremely traumatic and emotionally draining. The loss of reputation is a great concern and the fear of penalties or punishment paramount. Too often, when a charge is made against a practitioner, even before a proper investigation can be carried out, the case precipitates needlessly hasty publicity that implicates the practitioner and adds weight to the charge. This can do real harm to the good name of the practitioner and is unjust if the charge fails to be proved. The outcome of cases that are found in favour of the practitioner receive far less coverage than does the initial allegation. Too often people forget one of the premises of British law: that one is innocent until proven guilty.

Negligence is an aspect of the law of tort that comes under the general body of law known as the law of obligations. *Tort* is the French word for 'wrong' and it deals with the civil law of wrongdoing to another that is not serious enough to warrant a criminal proceeding but should be dealt with by some form of compensation to the injured party. Civil law is about solving disputes, negotiating settlements (as in family law matters and divorce proceedings) and compensating for breaches. Unlike criminal law, it does not seek to punish or rehabilitate an offender. Tort covers a wide range of topics. It includes breach of contract, actions against defamation/damage to reputation (favoured by celebrities), liability for defective premises as well as personal injury.

The development of tort is grounded in common law: the law that is made by the courts. Unlike the law made by an Act of Parliament that cannot be altered (unless a subsequent Act is written specifically to repeal it), laws that follow precedents set by a court ruling can change. New rulings can alter an existing precedent or set an entirely new one that is then followed until it is altered or amended in later cases. Hence, the tort of negligence, as applied to clinical practice, has evolved and continues to do so by rulings and decisions in seminal cases, most of which have dealt with medical cases but some of which come from entirely different situations (e.g. Donoghue v Stevenson [1932]; see below).

In our society, people are becoming more aware of their rights. Providers of products and services encourage customers, clients and patients to comment about the product and/or service they receive. This practice has led to people becoming more likely to complain and to demand some form of redress or compensation if they feel that they have been treated without adequate care or with substandard service. In health care, and particularly in medical practice, claims of negligence are rising. This does not mean that practitioners are becoming more careless, as many of the claims are not proved. It reflects the increasing likelihood of patients to make complaints against a practitioner when they feel dissatisfied with treatment or care.

Although a claim of negligence may be raised, this does not necessarily mean that it will succeed. For any charge of negligence to be proved, three essential conditions must be fulfilled:

1. There has to be a duty of care owed by one party to another.
2. The duty of care must have been breached.
3. Harm must have been suffered as a result of that breach of duty of care.

The onus of proof in a charge of negligence is on the person making the complaint.

THE DUTY OF CARE

The concept of a duty of care developed from one of the most famous cases in British law, and one that was seminal in the development of the modern law of tort: the case of Donoghue v Stevenson [1932]. This was not a case involving a practitioner and a patient, but about a young woman, a bottle of ginger beer and a snail. The case went to the (then) highest court in the land – the House of Lords – where Lord Atkin established his, now famous, 'neighbour' principle: that a person owes a duty of care to his or her neighbour (a neighbour being anyone who could be affected by one's actions). The concept of duty of care is now applied widely in the law of tort and is fundamental when dealing with the tort of negligence.

Donoghue v Stevenson [1932]

Miss Donoghue and a friend went into a shop/café for some refreshments. Miss Donoghue's friend ordered drinks. As part of the service, the shopkeeper opened a bottle of ginger beer for Miss Donoghue and poured part of it into a glass from which Miss Donoghue took a drink. Her friend subsequently poured the remaining contents of the bottle into the glass and found a decomposed snail floating out with the beverage. The bottle was made of dark glass, so it had not been possible to see the contents until they had been poured out. Miss Donoghue alleged that the decaying snail in her soft drink led to her becoming seriously ill and she subsequently sued Stevenson, the manufacturer of the drink, for negligence.

The case was complicated by the fact that the actions of Stevenson were not directly linked to Donoghue: a friend had bought the drink that was supplied by a shopkeeper who was selling Stevenson's products. Nevertheless, the courts found in favour of Miss Donoghue, and in the House of Lords one of the ruling Law Lords, Lord Atkin, put forward the principle that a duty of care is owed to anyone who may be affected or injured by an action or omission to act, if the effect of that action or omission on the injured party could reasonably be foreseen. Physical proximity between the wrongdoer and the injured was not necessary (Howarth & O'Sullivan 2000).

The ruling in Donoghue v Stevenson is considered to have established such a fundamental principle in tort that books on the law of tort often have a snail on the cover.

In healthcare practice, the first part of a claim for negligence, the duty of care, is not difficult to establish. Practitioners have a duty of care towards every patient that they see, treat and examine. In accordance with the 'neighbour' principle, they also have a broader duty of care to anyone with whom a patient may come into contact and who may be affected by negligent actions of the practitioner. A wrong prescription given to a patient may result in that patient having a car accident leading to a pedestrian being injured. The duty of care does not have to extend to all members of the public in all instances. A practitioner who witnesses an accident does not generally owe a duty of care to the victim. However, if he or she steps forward and declares their expertise, offering assistance as a practitioner, a duty of care is established.

There may be instances in which it is not clear how far a duty of care extends. For example, a practitioner has a private contract to conduct a series of clinical tests to screen patients for glaucoma and to look for factors that may be linked to increased intraocular pressure. The practitioner does not detect a cataract in one of the patients being screened. Whether or not the duty to screen for one condition extends to detection of another depends on whether the conditions are linked. If the cataract that was missed was a mature cataract and the lenticular swelling was a factor causing the increased intraocular pressure, the duty of care may extend to detecting the opacified lens and its impact on the intraocular pressure. If there was no link between the cataract and glaucoma, as the terms of service did not include cataract screening, the practitioner has not necessarily breached their duty of care.

Breach of duty of care

Once a duty of care has been established, the second part of a negligence claim requires proof that the practitioner has been in breach of an expected standard of care. In common law, many actions and behaviours are assessed against what can be expected of the 'ordinary reasonable' person. Because medical and healthcare practice requires a level of skill and expertise beyond that expected of an 'ordinary' person, the standard of care that a practitioner has to meet is also higher. This test for whether actions of a medical or healthcare practitioner have been negligent is known as the Bolam test, and is based on the direction given by the judge (Justice McNair) to the jury in the case of Bolam v Friern Hospital Management Committee [1957]:

> "The test is the standard of the ordinary skilled man exercising and professing to have that special skill."

Bolam v Friern Hospital Management Committee [1957]

John Bolam was a salesman who suffered from depression. He was seen by a psychiatrist and advised to undergo electroconvulsive therapy (ECT). The psychiatrist made no mention of the risks involved. Bolam was admitted to hospital the next day and signed a form consenting to the treatment. ECT was administered on two occasions by a senior registrar, and on the second it resulted in serious physical injuries to Bolam: dislocation of both hip joints and fractures of the pelvis. No relaxant drugs had been given to Bolam before the treatment and he was not restrained (apart from support to the lower jaw) during its administration. A charge of negligence was raised against the hospital for allowing the registrar to perform ECT without administering a relaxant drug before the treatment, for failing to provide proper restraint during treatment and for not warning the patient about the risks.

The body of medical opinion was divided on whether relaxant drugs should be given before ECT, whether there should be any physical restraint during treatment and whether patients should be warned of the risks. The risks of physical injuries of the types sustained by Bolam were said by experts to be extremely rare.

In his directions to the jury, the presiding judge Justice McNair stated that:

"A doctor is not guilty of negligence if he has acted in accordance with a practice accepted as proper by a responsible body of medical men skilled in that particular art."

The charge of negligence was not proved.

The Bolam test should not be misinterpreted as setting an absolute standard for practitioners. Neither does it expect a practitioner to work to the highest possible standards in their field. It is applied to determine whether a practitioner has been negligent by testing their actions against the standards of the ordinary practitioner. In other words, applying the Bolam test, if a practitioner is accused of negligence and other practitioners, specialized in the same field, say that what the accused did accorded with proper practice, the practitioner on trial is deemed not to be negligent. This applies even if a body of other practitioners has an alternative view on the matter.

Since Bolam, there has been another seminal case, Bolitho v City and Hackney Health Authority [1998], which modified the Bolam test by adding the proviso that the opinion of practitioners should be subject to logical analysis. Bolitho established the precedent that practitioners could not just give an opinion without substantiation and could not rely on a particular practice, as evidence against negligence, merely because it was established practice. The court had to be satisfied that the opinion had a sound and logical basis and that the practice was reasonable.

Bolitho v City and Hackney Health Authority [1998]

Patrick Bolitho was a 2-year-old boy admitted to hospital with breathing difficulties allegedly associated with croup, a condition caused by a virus and one that often clears spontaneously within a couple of days. The following day the child had breathing difficulties and the nurse called the doctor, but the doctor failed to attend. The child recovered but a couple of hours later had a recurrence of breathing problems; again the nurse called the doctor, who again did not come.

Shortly after this, the child suffered a cardiac arrest, and by the time cardiac function was restored Patrick was severely brain damaged. The parents brought a charge of negligence against the health authority, claiming that had the doctor attended when called, and had she intubated the child, the cardiac arrest and subsequent brain damage could have been prevented. Experts for both sides testified as to whether or not intubation could have saved the child. Opinions were divided. The doctor was found to be negligent for not attending but not responsible for causing the cardiac arrest and brain damage: the court accepted the opinion of an expert who claimed that intubation would not have helped the child.

Patrick Bolitho died before the end of legal proceedings.

The Bolitho modification established the principle that expert opinion is not necessarily the final determinant in deciding whether or not action taken or omission of an action by a practitioner could be considered as negligent. Although the Bolam test is still applied in cases of medical (clinical) negligence, there have been cases that showed that the court will be prepared to deviate from using it as the decisive test in determining whether or not a practitioner has been negligent. This was illustrated in the case of Smith v Tunbridge Wells Health Authority [1994] in which a patient brought a charge of negligence against the health authority because he had not been warned of the side-effects of surgery to repair a rectal prolapse. Experts testified that it was common and widely accepted practice not to tell patients about the side-effects of this type of surgery and, had the court applied the Bolam test, negligence would not have been found. Yet the court considered this practice irresponsible and unreasonable in spite of the fact that it accorded with the opinion of experts in the field. In the case of S (a woman with severe learning difficulties), the court ruled that, even if a treatment were established and agreed practice among practitioners/specialists, if it did not accord with the best interests of the patient, the latter should be the paramount in deciding a course of action (Re S [2001]).

To determine whether a practitioner has breached his or her duty of care to a patient, the law will depend on the opinion of other practitioners and measure against the standards expected of the ordinary practitioner. The courts will subject the opinions of experts to logical analysis, and the best interests of the patient will be considered.

Harm was suffered as a result of the breach

The final part of a negligence claim deals with whether the breach of duty of care by the practitioner resulted in the harm or injury that led to the negligence claim. This can be the hardest aspect of negligence to prove and many claims fail because of a failure to link the breach of duty of care with the harm or injury sustained. The case of Bolitho is an example of this: although the doctor was found to have breached her duty of care by not attending the patient when called, the non-attendance was not found to have caused the damage suffered.

To establish a link between the practitioner's actions or inactions and the damage to the patient, requires investigation of two aspects of the harm/injury: causation and remoteness.

Causation

This is often referred to, in legal textbooks, as 'factual causation', indicating that the law seeks to the look at whether the facts show the injury or damage to have been caused by the practitioner. Commonly the courts use what is called the 'but for' test, i.e. the injury would not have occurred *but for* the breach of duty of care by the practitioner. In other words, had the practitioner not acted as they did, there would have been no harm or injury. The 'but for' test is relatively stringent and requires the person who is making the claim to prove that the actions of the person against whom the claim is made directly caused the injury or harm. If the actions of anyone else or a chain of other events contributed to the injury, so much so that it could not be said with certainty that the practitioner's action caused the injury, the claim of negligence against the practitioner is likely to fail.

Recently there has been a relaxation in the strict application of this test in cases where there could be only one causal factor. In the case of Fairchild v Glenhaven Funeral Services Ltd and Others [2002], employees had worked for more than one employer and had not been protected against the inhalation of asbestos dust by either employer. Application of the 'but for' test would have been very difficult to prove against either employer, because it would require proving that the actions of one or other employer caused the harm. Because there was a single cause of harm, the use of asbestos, and the employee would not have been able to distinguish the effects of asbestos on his health from one employer or another, application of the 'but for' test would mean that the claim would fail and neither employer would be found negligent. Indeed, this is what happened at the Court of Appeal. The claim proceeded to a higher court and the House of Lords felt that it would not be in the interests of justice to adhere to the 'but for' test when it was clear that asbestos dust was the only cause of the harm and that both employers had acted negligently. It was not important which one was the more negligent, and both employers were found to be liable.

A single cause brought about by more than one practitioner could occur in clinical practice if two or more practitioners were negligent in the treatment of the patient in exactly the same way. For example, two practitioners consecutively fail to diagnose giant papillary conjunctivitis in a contact lens-wearing patient who presents with symptoms of sore eyes and irritation, and both advise the patient to persist with the lenses.

The 'but for' test can be applied effectively if there is a simple cause-and-effect link: a practitioner provides a patient with spectacles of the wrong prescription and the patient, unable to see clearly through the spectacles, trips, falls and is injured. The situation can be complicated when there are a number of possible causes.

Clinical case study

Mr Jones presents for an eye examination complaining of sore, red eyes, and says that the pain started the day before. There is a family history of glaucoma, and examination shows that intraocular pressures are more than 30 mmHg and the pupils are slightly oval shaped. Mr Jones is asked to sit in the waiting room; he is told that he will need to see a specialist at the hospital and that the practitioner will arrange for this immediately. Mr Jones goes back to the waiting room and his wife asks about the outcome of the examination. He tells her that he has been told to wait for another 'specialist'. The receptionist comes in and calls out the name of 'Mr Johns'. Her voice is neither clear nor loud, and Mr Jones and his wife mishear it as 'Mr Jones'. Mr Jones steps forward. (Mr Johns, who was waiting for an ophthalmoscopic examination, has just gone out of the building for a cigarette.) The receptionist asks Mr Jones to go into a particular examination room where the practice nurse is waiting to put a drop into his eye. The nurse instills a mydriatic drop in Mr Jones' right eye and then tells him to return to the waiting room for about 20 minutes, after which he will be called for a further examination.

Mr Jones suffers an attack of glaucoma and subsequent sight loss.

Who has been negligent and whose actions have caused the damage:

- *The practitioner – for not ensuring that the patient had properly understood that he was about to be referred to a specialist at the hospital and that he needed to wait for a letter to be prepared and not for a further examination at the practice?*
- *The nurse – for not attempting to identify the patient properly before instilling the drops in his eye?*
- *The receptionist – for not being clear in calling out the patient's name and not checking his details against a record card?*
- *The patient – for not listening to the practitioner properly?*

If this case proceeded to court, such questions would arise in trying to establish causation. The receptionist could not be held responsible for medical negligence as she has no duty of care as a practitioner to a patient. However, as her actions could have added to precipitating the harm, the causal links between the harm and the actions of the practitioner and the nurse could be deemed to be more tenuous. The practitioner could also be vicariously liable for the actions of the receptionist (discussed later).

When injury or harm occurs as a result of a number of contributory causes, it can be difficult to determine whether there is one predominant cause and whether or not the actions of a single person could, alone, have led to the harm. Courts faced with such a situation look to the question of remoteness: how remote were the actions of the person against whom the charge of negligence is made, from the actual harm that occurred?

Remoteness

Once it has been established that there was a causal link between the breach of the duty of care and the resultant injury or harm, the law considers the extent of the liability in negligence. The law does not assume that, just because it has been proved that there has been a breach of duty of care and that this led to injury or harm, this means the person accused of the breach should be held responsible for the full extent of the injury or harm. In a clinical context, the law considers how much blame can be placed on a practitioner who has breached their duty of care to a patient where the breach has resulted in some injury or harm. The degree of liability of a practitioner is established by considering the 'remoteness' of his or her actions from the injury.

To investigate the extent of liability or remoteness of harm or injury, the courts apply the test of 'forseeability': could the practitioner have foreseen that his or her actions would lead to the injury or harm caused to the patient? This test was established in a case of The Wagon Mound [1961], in which oil was negligently spilled from a tanker in Sydney Harbour and led to a fire that destroyed ships and part of the dock. A more recent case has emphasized that it is not necessary to forsee the severity of the injury or harm, or exactly how it could occur, in order to be deemed liable for negligence (Jolley v Sutton Borough Council [2000]).

What this means for a practitioner is that, if it can be shown that they should have foreseen that their actions would cause injury or harm to the patient, they will not be considered too remote from the damage and would be held liable for its full extent. Conversely, even if a practitioner has breached his or her duty of care, if it is held by the court that the harm or injury that occurred could not have been forseen, the court may dismiss a claim of negligence.

POTENTIAL FOR NEGLIGENCE IN PRIMARY EYE CARE PRACTICE

The cases that may be the most likely to invoke a claim of negligence are those in which serious and/or sustained damage to sight has occurred.

Causing an injury

The most likely cause of direct injury is by contact tonometry. This may have an immediate effect if epithelial cell damage is substantial enough to cause pain and possibly some blurring of vision. Superficial corneal scarring, however, usually heals relatively quickly with no ensuing loss of sight. If the patient tries to claim that an injury, caused by contact tonometry, led to an infection that occurred months later, such a claim could be very difficult to prove.

Not informing a patient about a condition

Good practitioners will inform patients about ocular disease or conditions that need treatment or particular care. Not informing a patient about a serious or progressive condition that subsequently leads to loss of sight can lead to a claim of negligence. However, there are situations in which the condition is not detrimental to vision, does not require any immediate attention, and the practitioner may consider that telling the patient about it may cause unnecessary alarm.

A common example of this is early cataract. In the past it was common practice not to mention the presence of a cataract to a patient if the opacification of the lens was not causing any significant problems with vision and there was no need for an operation. Recently, practitioners have been encouraged to be more open with patients, and patients have come to expect this. Just how open and frank cannot be given with certainty because practitioners must have some discretion in what they consider a patient should be told. The variations in what is communicated could result in a situation in which a patient is not told by one practitioner about the presence of early cataracts but learns about this from another practitioner. If such a patient were to claim negligence against the first practitioner, the claim would fail because, even if not informing a patient about the presence of early cataract is considered to be a breach of duty of care, there would have been no harm or injury resulting from this breach. A cataract does not progress so rapidly that an early warning and immediate intervention is required.

Failing to diagnose a serious disease or condition

Retinal detachments, glaucoma and tumours are examples of conditions that require immediate attention. Misdiagnosing or missing vital signs and symptoms of such conditions could lead to a claim of negligence. Patients with retinal detachments can present describing strange symptoms or fail to mention any at all. Tumours can present in different forms and may be mistaken for ordinary pigmentation. A primary care practitioner may not be expected to diagnose a tumour but, in the best interests of the patient, should refer any unusual signs to a specialist.

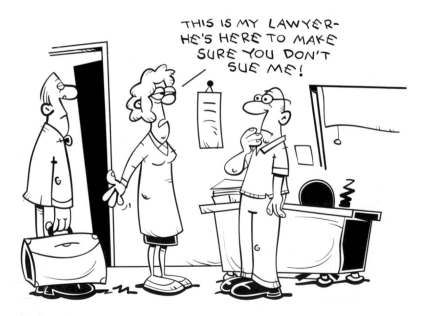

CLAIMS FOR DAMAGES AND PRACTITIONER PROTECTION

A patient who can prove negligence against a practitioner will be compensated in the form of damages payment; the amount is decided by a judge if the matter goes to court. Out of court settlements are decided between parties, generally negotiated through the respective legal representatives. Insurance should cover much of the financial cost. The cost to reputation, health and well-being of the practitioner cannot be as easily recovered. Practitioners should not yield to patients who are merely seeking compensation when no harm has occurred. The 'vexatious litigant' is thankfully rare but, when one does appear, such a patient should not be appeased with monetary compensation if the complaint is without substance. No practitioner should have to suffer a loss of reputation, earnings or emotional distress because a patient is making unreasonable demands or false accusations. The respect and understanding that a practitioner gives a patient should be reciprocated, and practitioners have a right to expect it. Unfortunately, there are no ethical guidelines for patients to follow because ethics is the domain of a professional group. The profession should be more active in protecting the practitioner against such patients, and colleagues should be prepared to support a practitioner who is falsely or unfairly accused of negligence or malpractice.

THE IMPORTANCE OF KEEPING RELIABLE RECORDS

If a claim is made against a practitioner, the strength of the practitioner's defence will rely crucially on the clinical record. A practitioner who only has his or her verbal evidence against the word of a patient will be in a weaker position than the patient, because a patient is not expected to keep a written record. Records that show careful reasoned notes, consistency and order indicate that the practitioner is organized and that his or her evidence is dependable.

It is somewhat sad that practitioners are advised to think defensively (i.e. to consider how the record would stand up to scrutiny in a court or tribunal proceeding) when they are recording observations made and what has been said to and by patients (Warburton 2004).

Defensive thinking suggests that the practitioner needs continually to be prepared for the possibility that a patient may make a complaint, and this would appear to be contrary to building up a bond of mutual trust between patient and practitioner. It is, however, advice to be heeded. In the current clime of patients' rights and charters, and the ever greater measures taken to 'protect' the patient, defensive thinking is both wise and necessary for the protection of the practitioner.

Although it would be unreasonable to expect a practitioner to prepare an entire transcript of a consultation, the following should always be considered when recording what was done or said:

- Tests that were conducted, why the tests were conducted and what equipment was used, for example: 'The eye was dilated because symptoms of retinal detachment were reported; both direct and indirect ophthalmoscopy were used.'
- Why a particular test may not have been done; for example, in a patient who shows signs and symptoms of glaucoma but also has Parkinson's disease and cannot keep his head still, a visual field test would not be reliable. This should be recorded.
- Record the findings of normal as well as of abnormal signs. If the fundus of a diabetic patient has no signs of the disease, this should be noted as it indicates that the test was conducted. No recording could, and in a tribunal or court hearing probably would, be interpreted as an indication that the test was not done.
- Interpretation of what the observations may be indicating and what the practitioner thinks they may not be indicating. This can help to explain why certain tests were not conducted. For example, if a practitioner decides that a patient with a red eye is suffering from an infection of the anterior eye and glaucoma has been ruled out, not taking intraocular pressure readings with a contact tonometer can be justified.
- Records should always be clear and comprehensible. A practitioner who treats the patient at a later date must be able to understand the medical history of the patient. Shorthand notations or illegible handwriting are not only difficult for other practitioners to understand, they may be deemed unacceptable as evidence in a court or tribunal hearing.
- Patients should be given good, clear explanations of everything that was done or why it may be necessary, and the record should testify to this. Noting that an explanation has been given and what was said and that the patient has understood is an indication that

the communication has taken place. If, at a later date, the patient denies being informed about a treatment or procedure (and this may be because the patient has forgotten), the practitioner can point to the record. With serious conditions and where the practitioner may have reservations that the patient is listening or may not feel comfortable about the patient's reliability to remember, it may even be helpful to have the patient sign that an explanation has been given and that the patient has understood it. It is also worth recording a patient's response to advice or to an explanation. If the patient expresses agreement and even enthusiasm for a certain treatment and returns subsequently to say that they were opposed to it from the start, a record showing prior consent is the best means of defence. Practitioners need to be prepared that patients may forget what they are told. Research has shown how unreliable patient recollection or understanding of procedures can be.

Patient recollections

- One study found that 2–5 days after an operation, 27% of patients did not know on which organ surgery had been undertaken and 44% were unaware of the basic facts relating to the operation (Byrne et al 1988).
- A study of 100 patients receiving chemotherapy, who were given written information about the therapy and had signed a consent form permitting it to be administered, found that:

    (a) only 34 patients understood the purpose of the form and only one considered it to be a major source of information;
    (b) 75 patients could not name any of their drugs;
    (c) 26 patients did not know the aim of the therapy; and
    (d) only 15 patients remembered all four side-effects (Olver et al 1995).

- Another study found that 69% of patients admitted that they had not read the consent form before signing it, although those who had read the form were not significantly better informed than those who did not do so (Lavelle-Jones et al 1993).

- If a practitioner recommends a course of action and the patient refuses to take this advice, the patient should be asked to sign a written statement indicating that the recommendation was given by the practitioner but that the patient refused it.

- Whether or not a patient presents for an examination should be recorded. Warburton (2004) points out that a patient may be confused about which practice they attended. If a patient insists that an examination took place and the appointments book confirms that an appointment was made for that time and date, the records show no evidence of an examination (because the patient did not, in fact, attend), but no note is made of non-attendance, there is little to defend the practitioner.

Record retention

There is no specified ruling about record retention, only recommendations that can vary with time. Currently, the Department of Health recommends that hospital records be kept for 10 years, and for children record retention should be until the child reaches 25 years of age, or 26 years if treatment was concluded at the age of 17 years; if the child dies before reaching the age of 18 years, the record should be kept for 8 years after death (Department of Health 2006). The College of Optometrists (2007) recommends following the National Health Service (NHS) guidelines. The Association of Optometrists (AOP) recommends that records of adult patients seen in private practice should be retained for 12 years, records of children until the age of 25 years and for at least 12 years after the last visit, and records of the deceased for 10 years (Warburton 2004).

Excessively long retention of records would be contrary to the fifth principle of the Data Protection Act 1998, which stipulates that personal data should not be kept longer than necessary for the purpose for which it was collected. However, what is 'necessary for purpose' depends on the patient and the length of time that the patient continues to belong to a particular practice. A young person who becomes a patient at the age of 12 years, has a chronic condition and continues to be a patient at the same practice into late adulthood may have a record dating back over decades, with justification.

When considering record retention, for the purposes of protection against a claim in negligence, what needs to be taken into account is the limitation period for pursuing a valid claim. In other words, how long does a patient have to make a claim before it is invalidated by the passage of time? The Limitation Act 1980 stipulates that a claim has to be made within 3 years of the date of the injury or 3 years from the date that a realization of the injury is made by the person bringing the claim (s11 Limitation Act 1980). This means that, if a patient is made aware 2 years after treatment has finished that the treatment may have caused the injury or harm that the patient is suffering, the limitation period of 3 years starts from the date that the patient realized that there may be a causal connection. In such a case the patient can make a claim up to 5 years after the treatment was provided. For minors, the limitation period does not start until they reach the age of 18 years, and there is a provision in section 33 of the Limitation Act 1980 that gives a court discretion to allow a claim beyond the 3-year statutory limitation period.

Hence, although there is a specified limitation period, the commencement of this period can vary and be varied. Practitioners are therefore advised to retain records and be insured. Insurance is now a mandatory condition of registration, and the retired practitioner should maintain some form of insurance for several years after retirement.

VICARIOUS LIABILITY

Practitioners can be held vicariously liable for the negligence of their non-optometric staff. A cautionary example of this was cited in the NHS Litigation Authority Journal (Hepworth 2005). A patient, who was blind in one eye, noticed a clouding in the functional eye. She immediately phoned her general practitioner (GP), only to be told by the receptionist that there were no appointments available. The receptionist suggested that the patient should see an optometrist. The patient took this advice and, the following day, was seen by an optometrist.

The optometrist's findings suggested that there was a retinal detachment in that eye and a note was written to the GP asking for immediate referral of the patient to a hospital. The patient phoned the GP surgery for an immediate appointment and was again told there were none available. She promptly went to another GP practice, registered there, was seen immediately and was referred to hospital. After the operation the patient was left with 30–40% vision and the consultant ophthalmologist said that some of this sight loss could be attributed to the delay in being seen and referred. The patient took action against the first GP with whom she had had no contact. The GP had not even been aware that the patient had tried to contact her. Although culpability was entirely that of the receptionist, and it was recognized in the tribunal that the GP was not aware of how the receptionist had behaved, the GP was held vicariously liable for the actions of the receptionist. A receptionist, who has no duty of care to a patient, cannot be held responsible for negligence, so the liability passes to the practitioner.

Support staff should be trained to be alert for patients who request urgent treatment and for the types of descriptors that may justify an immediate examination (e.g. flashing lights, floaters, sudden loss or impairment of vision). Provision should always be made to see these patients.

SUMMARY

Negligence in clinical practice requires proof that the duty of care that a practitioner has to a patient has been breached and that the breach resulted in harm or injury. Case law has set precedents for what is required to prove negligence. One of the most important means of defence for a practitioner who has been accused of negligence is the patient record. Records need to be thorough, complete and retained for sufficient periods. Practitioners ought to be aware that claims can be made years after the patient has been seen and that they may be vicariously liable for their non-clinical staff.

References

Bolam v Friern Hospital Management Committee, Queen's Bench Division [1957] 2 All ER 118, [1957] 1 WLR 582, 1 BMLR 1

Bolitho v City and Hackney Health Authority [1998] AC 232

Byrne D J, Napier A, Cuschieri A 1988 How informed is signed consent? British Medical Journal 296:839–840

College of Optometrists 2007 Code of ethics and guidelines for professional conduct. Section 35: Patient records. Online. Available: http://www.college-optometrists.org/index.aspx/pcms/site.publication.Ethics_Guidelines.recent/

Data Protection Act 1998 Online. Available: http://www.opsi.gov.uk/ACTS/acts1998/19980029.htm

Department of Health 2006 Records management: NHS code of practice. Part 2, Annex D1. Online. Available: http://www.dh.gov.uk/en/Publicationsandstatistics/Publications/PublicationsPolicyAndGuidance/DH_4131747

Donoghue v Stevenson [1932] AC 562; [1932] HL All ER Rep 1

Fairchild v Glenhaven Funeral Services Ltd and Others [2002] UKHL 22; Fox v Spousal (Midlands) Ltd; Matthews v Associated Portland Cement Manufacturers (1978) Ltd and Another [2002] ICR 798B

Hepworth S (ed.) 2005 Urgent appointment refused. Case cited in the NHS Litigation Authority Journal 4:12–13; also cited in the South Gloucestershire Primary Care Trust Clinical Governance Newsletter June 2005, Issue No. 6. Online. Available: http://www.sglos-pct.nhs. uk/ClinGov/newsletters/June%202005%20Issue%206.pdf

Howarth D R, O'Sullivan J A 2000 Hepple, Howarth and Matthews' tort: cases and materials, 5th edn. Butterworths, London

Jolley v Sutton Borough Council [2000] 1 WLR 1082

Lavelle-Jones C, Byrne D J, Rice P, Cuschieri A 1993 Factors affecting quality of informed consent. British Medical Journal 306:885–890

Limitation Act 1980 The UK Statute Law Database. Online. Available: http://www.statutelaw.gov.uk/

Olver I N, Buchanan L, Laidlaw C, Poulton G 1995 The adequacy of consent forms for informing patients entering oncological clinical trials. Annals of Oncology 6:867–870

Re S (Adult Patient Sterilisation) [2001] 2 Fam 15

Smith v Tunbridge Wells Health Authority [1994] 5 Med LR 334

The Wagon Mound [1961] AC 388(PC)

Warburton T 2004 Litigation and record keeping. Better to be safe than sorry. Optometry Today 20 August:20–23

10

Business ethics

THE ESSENCE OF BUSINESS

There is no denying that the prime objective of business is to make a monetary gain. To some people this is perfectly acceptable as long as the means of creating wealth are honest and fair. To others the idea that 'making money' is an aim in itself is disturbing; a certain amount of money is needed to sustain a reasonable lifestyle, but to generate excess wealth and to have this as a major objective seems somehow wrong. These people generally have a keen sense of the inequalities in our world, the starving masses in continents such as Africa compared and contrasted to what have been labelled as 'obscenely' rich magnates who think nothing about spending millions of pounds or dollars on a party. Somewhere between the extremes of making a profit for the sake of funding an excessively lavish lifestyle and generating only enough income to cover the needs for a basic life there are ways of running a successful and highly ethical business.

To some eye care practitioners, those who work in hospitals or for public bodies, the ethics of business may not be particularly pertinent. To those who work in private practice, running a business is an integral part of working life because, alongside offering a healthcare service, the practitioner is selling a product. Indeed, in private practice, the greater share of the profits comes from the sale of spectacles, contact lenses and other aids to vision than it does from the provision of health care. Reconciling the business and the healthcare provision aspects of private practice requires that a comfortable balance be reached between the two. How this balance is achieved depends on the practitioner, the perspective he or she has on healthcare practice and its place in society and, fundamentally, how the practitioner treats those whom he or she serves.

THE ROOTS OF BUSINESS ETHICS

An interest in business ethics is neither new nor recent but can be traced back, as far as the Western world is concerned, over seven centuries (Vogel 1991). Great theologians, philosophers and thinkers have contributed views on the morality and ethics of business. Notably, the conflict between profit and ethical practice has been debated and examined extensively. There was a time when business and ethics were considered mutually exclusive. Treating profit-making as morally reprehensible could, understandably, be justified when business practice (as in medieval times) included placing animal carcasses in the shops of opponent merchants to stymie competition by making the employees and customers sick (Vogel 1991). The attitude of the Church in medieval times was that profit-making was not a moral activity and as such it could hardly be considered ethical. The emergence of Protestant thought during the Reformation, that considered money as an accepted reward for work, altered the attitude to business. If a job was done well and with honesty there was nothing immoral or unethical about gaining from it financially. Over the centuries, questions of morality and ethics in business practice have resurfaced and currently business ethics is a growing subject. Vogel (1991) points out that, although current interest in business ethics is concerned with organizations, and the notion of social responsibility of corporations, rather than, as in the past, with the behaviour and character of individuals, the basic dilemmas remain the same. In terms of health care, the balance between business and ethics is even more sensitive because the customer is the patient.

PATIENT OR CUSTOMER: COMMERCE OR CONSULTATION

A patient presents for help or advice on health; a customer comes for a product. A patient should never been seen as a means of making a profit; a customer is often portrayed in this way. It is easy to reconcile profit-making with product sales; indeed, in the business world the two are often equated. This can be done because a sale is a quantifiable transaction: a sum of money is exchanged for a particular product and, if two such products are purchased, the sum of money paid is generally doubled (unless a discount is offered). This is not the same with healthcare provision and in the treatment of patients. No two patients are alike and payment is not made strictly on the basis of what is provided: the practitioner does not charge per minute of case history taking, per tests conducted, per treatment advised. If this was the means by which practitioners were paid for healthcare provision, immediate inequalities would arise: the poor could not afford as much of the practitioner's time or to have as many tests conducted. Practitioners could tailor treatment so that they could optimize the money to be made and this could lead to unethical practice. Health care clearly cannot operate entirely as a business venture, but this does not mean that aspects of practice that involve product sales should avoid profit as an objective. The sale of the product can be seen as assisting the healthcare provision, but should not become the primary purpose of practice.

The degree of emphasis on the commercial side of practice varies depending on practice type. A practitioner who works in a small practice, is self-employed or in partnership with others can determine how much time is given per consultation, may wish to introduce specialized practice and may be relatively flexible in the way that the sale of spectacles, contact lenses or appliances are managed. Working for an independent group of practitioners may allow less flexibility in the management of sales: practices from the same group may require similar consultation periods, compare patient output, provide the same offers and discounts, stock the same spectacles, deal with the same suppliers. The larger the scale of the business, the less flexible, for each individual practitioner, may be the commercial as well as the consultative aspects.

PATIENT CHOICE

In addition to the dichotomy, from the point of view of the practitioner, between the business and the treatment aspects of healthcare practice, there are changes within the healthcare sector that are affecting how patients see healthcare provision. With the increase in managerial posts within the National Health Service (NHS) and an increasing emphasis on patients having a greater say in their own treatment, healthcare provision appears to be shifting from the hands of the practitioners, to patients, administrators and ultimately to market forces. The debate about the impact of market forces and competition in health care has concentrated on medical practice but is no less relevant to other areas of health care. On the one hand, competition and a market-based approach can be considered as improving healthcare provision because the market responds to the consumer and hence becomes more efficient (Enthoven 1985, cited by Fitzgerald & Ferlie 2000). The opposing argument is that market forces can be instrumental in a degeneration of collegiality and a fragmentation of the bonds that link practitioners (Hafferty 1988, cited by Fitzgerald & Ferlie 2000). This would lead to a deterioration of trust and ethical behaviour towards fellow practitioners. How people treat others with whom they interact, whether in personal/social life or in the workplace, depends on individual personality traits, personal principles and ethics as well as on ambitions.

Patient choice, nevertheless, cannot be the same as consumer choice. Sale of products depends on their popularity and consequent demand and this may have little to do with product worth, durability or any benefit it may bring to the purchaser or to society as a whole. Demand is often based on an emerging and sometimes short-lived trend. The sale of ever-newer mobile phone models and accompanying ring-tones are two examples. Treatment of illnesses, conditions and diseases does not follow popular trends or provide the wide choice seen with product sales. It is limited not only by what is available but also by what is appropriate. Even when appropriate treatment is provided, a complete guarantee that it will meet the need or desire of the patient cannot be given. The patient who chooses laser eye surgery to correct myopia cannot be assured that every excess dioptre will be corrected. The final refraction depends on factors that can and cannot be controlled, such as healing of the cornea, and some residual myopia may remain. In cases of chronic or terminal conditions, treatment may go only as far as alleviating pain and prolonging life. Often there may be unpleasant side-effects. Patients generally understand this and do not demand the same complete satisfaction with treatment as with the purchase of a product.

There is also the factor of cost. Whilst the customer or consumer pays for whatever they wish to purchase, healthcare provision, unless it involves private treatment, is paid for by the government with contributions from all tax-paying individuals. What is provided to the patient is, therefore, regulated by the government. Even with the increase in patient choice and influence, as long as health care is paid for from the public purse, availability will depend on what the government prioritizes as giving the most benefit to the greatest number of patients.

MANAGEMENT ETHICS AND SOCIAL RESPONSIBILITY

Business involves the management of people, and management styles vary depending on the individual. A style of management that is Machiavellian was adopted in the past and excused on the basis that it was efficient. It involved a manipulation of other people, distortion of truth and exploitation in order to gain power and control: self-interest was the predominant driving force.

Management

"Power is the proximal cause of leadership and the precursor of success in management. For the manager there are two basic challenges in leading a group. The first is gaining control; the second is keeping it."

(From Griffin 1991)

There is no doubt that this management style is still employed and it is acknowledged that some people in management positions have a natural tendency to behave without any regard to ethics (Beu et al 2003). Indeed, there are people who occupy powerful positions and have reached these through purely Machiavellian means, but it is becoming no longer acceptable for such behaviour to continue in the workplace. Beu et al (2003) make the point that for business to function it must adopt the norms of society in terms of behaviour and an understanding of what is right and what is wrong. Profit-making is therefore acceptable as long as it fits in with values of fair treatment of others, equality of opportunity, honesty and trust. Climbing the ladder of success and achievement at work is not wrong as long it does not involve treading on and harming others to ensure a swifter elevation. Ethical practice is now an integral part of business and management, and the teaching of ethics has been advocated as an essential part of all MBA courses (Block & Cwik 2007).

The importance and role of ethics in business are viewed with varying perspectives, and the arguments about how much social responsibility a business is obliged to accept are wide. Early reasoning by Friedman (1970) would appear to concur, to some extent, with the Machiavellian model, if money and power are equated, for Friedman rejects any notion of social responsibility stating that managers should focus solely on profit-making and wealth maximization for the business or organization. Following Friedman's argument, employees should renounce their own ethics, beliefs and values, once in the workplace, if these contradict expected standards of the organization (Mudrack 2007). The opposing argument is that the organization or business cannot be treated as the major or sole stakeholder: employees and those whom they may serve should also be considered and may, at times, be more important that the interests of the business (Mudrack 2007). Whatever view is held depends on the approach of the individual to management and to the concept of fairness and equity. Mason & Mudrack (1997) have reported that social traditionalists – those who would support Friedman's view on social responsibility – also tend to have a Machiavellian personality type and feel that it is more equitable to receive rather than to give. These individuals pay little regard to ethics and have a distrust of the motives of others (Mudrack 2007). Those with a greater regard for social responsibility consider the interests of others and have a more universal concept of fairness and equity.

Whilst it is accepted that personalities and outlooks will vary, caution is advised when considering putting a social traditionalist with Machiavellian views into a management position. Clearly, when dealing with patients, practitioners are expected to put self-interest aside and apply ethical principles to clinical practice, but a practitioner who is also the manager of a practice, and therefore responsible for the business aspects, ought to apply similar ethical attitudes to colleagues, other employees and subordinates. If an individual cannot manage with consideration for others, that individual is not suited to a management role. Ethics should never be sacrificed for self-interest and monetary gain.

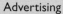

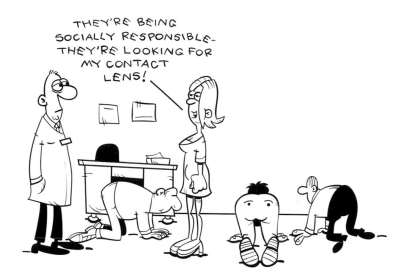

ADVERTISING

For many people, there is a lingering doubt about whether or not advertising can ever be an ethical activity. Yet, advertising is an integral part of selling in the business world (as we know it) and hence if advertising is unethical so, *de facto*, is business. To understand why advertising has such a dubious reputation requires a consideration of how its role in business is perceived. Klempner (2006) categorizes the arguments commonly cited against those who advertise, into three 'charges':

1. that it *sells dreams* and therefore confuses reality with fantasy;
2. that is *panders* to desire for things that may not promote good;
3. that it *manipulates* people into buying what they do not need.

These accusations suggest that advertising deliberately deceives, promotes hedonism and encourages wastefulness. Yet, Klempner (2006) defends advertising by arguing that dreams are a part of the reality of living and that, as long as advertising does not sell dreams that can never be realized and does not offer false hope, it does not deceive and should not necessarily be deemed unethical. Whatever product or service is being advertised, it should not have been created with money-making as its sole aim.

In healthcare practice, advertising a service or product cannot ever be deemed as selling a dream. It is not a purely profit-building exercise. Patients may respond to an advertisement but they do not come into a practice because they are enticed by the idea of an eye examination; they come in when they perceive a need for advice, treatment, regular monitoring, reassurance. What is gained by the service is, primarily, a benefit to the health of the patient. If services rendered, in time, bring the practitioner a measure of wealth, as long as the service has been properly provided and honestly advertised, any wealth is rightfully earned and advertising the service should not be considered unethical.

The charge of pandering to desires has been levelled at elective or cosmetic surgery techniques. They are regarded by some practitioners and non-practitioners as not only unnecessary but also unethical because they expose a patient to risks that cannot be justified on the grounds of health promotion or disease prevention. Laser surgery to correct refractive errors is not a sight-saving procedure, nor is it the only or necessarily the best treatment available for refractive correction. It carries the greatest risk and is the most expensive. Advertising such a procedure is viewed, by those who oppose it, as promoting unethical practice. However, a patient who deplores the wearing of spectacles and cannot wear contact lenses may consider laser surgery as the only option. In such a case, the effect of the procedure on the well-being of the patient may be so great that it brings genuine benefits to the health of the patient. The respect for patient choice and autonomy supports ethical practice. As long as a patient is not coerced into having the surgery and the advertising is not deceptive, there are valid arguments against treating such procedures and their advertising as unethical.

Advertising spectacle frames or contact lenses is similar to the advertising of any product: it appeals to aesthetics, it uses beautiful models and it suggests that the product will enhance the appearance of the wearer. Whether or not this is manipulative is debatable. As spectacles are generally worn by individuals who need refractive correction, it would be erroneous to argue that the advertising of spectacle frames manipulates people to buy what they do not need. The charge of manipulation can perhaps be raised in relation to the cost of frames: that advertising entices a patient to buy a more expensive frame when a cheaper one would do. This argument, however, supports depriving the patient of choice. The right of a person to choose their own style, whether this applies to choice of dress (provided it is not offensive) or to choice of frames, should be respected. Advertising, in this case, showcases and promotes choice and, as such, it is difficult to call such advertising unethical.

Case study

George is an established optometrist in a large town. He has an excellent reputation and comes from a family of optometrists who have provided eye care service to the town and surrounding regions for three generations. Over this time the town has grown and so has the family practice. Bill is a more recent graduate who has decided to set up a small optometric practice on the other side of the town. George has welcomed Bill and given him helpful advice about setting up a practice, aspects of patient care, dealing with suppliers, the locality and the types of patients he may expect to see. One day Bill approaches George to ask about the best way to advertise his practice more widely and how he should compose and design the advertisement. George smiles at Bill and says: 'I am happy to give you advice on practice-based matters and health care, but not when it comes to advertising. You are asking me to help you in competing with me. That would be, for me, a conflict of interests."

Is George being fair? How far should collegiality extend in business?

CONTRACT LAW

A fundamental aspect of business is a contractual obligation. Relationships and transactions are regulated by contracts. In its simplest form a contract can be represented by the following simple equation:

$$OFFER + ACCEPTANCE = CONTRACT$$

One party makes an offer and the party to whom it is made accepts the offer. A contract is formed. A common misconception is that a contract is valid only if it is made in writing and signed. In fact, a legally binding contract can be made via oral communication or by conduct. It is, of course, much more difficult to prove a breach of contract if there is no written agreement, but it is nonetheless recognized in law.

The offer can be made to a person, to a group of people, or even to the 'whole world'. The inclusion of the 'whole world' as a group to whom an offer can be made arose from a seminal case dating back over a century, in which a company advertised their product in such a way that an offer was seen to have been included in the advertisement.

An offer to the whole world

Carbolic Smoke Ball Company put out an advertisement to the public stating that they were so sure of their product as a protection against influenza that they would pay £100 to any person who took their medication (the smoke ball) and contracted influenza after taking it. Mrs Carlill bought the medication, took it as prescribed and subsequently became ill with influenza. When she sued Carbolic Smoke Ball for £100, the company argued that this could not have been a contract or a valid offer because it was made to the 'whole world' and this would be impossible in law. The court ruled that it was in fact possible to make an offer to the whole world, sending a clear message to any advertisers who may attempt to use a scam offer as an inducement to buy their product. (From the case of Carlill v Carbolic Smoke Ball Company [1893].)

In the context of eye care practice, if a manufacturer of frames adds to their advertising material the claim that these frames are made to last for 5 years regardless of how they are treated and backs the claim with a full money-back offer, this would have to be honoured in the event of a breakage. An advertisement is not itself an offer but if the advertisement contains a promise to do something, this promise can constitute an offer and must be honoured to avoid breach of contract. Advertising a reward in return for a member of the public finding something that has been lost can also be considered as an offer.

In addition to the agreement between the person who has made the offer and the one who has accepted it, in order for a contract to be legally binding, it must have:

- validity
- consideration
- intention.

The offer and the acceptance must be valid; in other words, it must be able to be made and accepted. It is not valid to offer to sell something belonging to someone else or something that was illegally acquired (stolen goods, drugs). A valid acceptance can be made only if the offer is still in force (it has not lapsed), the acceptance is by the person to whom the offer was made and there is an acceptance on the same terms as those stated in the offer. Many disputes arise because an offer is made on one set of terms and the acceptance is made on the basis of another.

Consideration means 'something for something': one party offers to give another something of value or benefit in exchange for some form of remuneration or other means of payment. An offer to drive a colleague into work, which is duly accepted, cannot form a contract because the colleague is not giving back anything that may be considered of value (the pleasure of the person's company does not constitute value in the eyes of the law).

Finally there has to be an intention on the part of both parties to a contract that they wish to enter into it. A contract is not valid if a party has been forced, coerced or deceived into making the agreement.

The agreement that is made in the contract will contain some form of undertaking by the parties to the agreement. These undertakings are the terms of the contract and if they are stated (in an oral contract) or written (in a document) they are called express terms. Such terms describe the obligations of all parties to a contract and what can happen in the event of a breach. Often, a contract also contains implied terms: those not stipulated but expected by law to be fulfilled in order for the contract to be efficacious. For example, expecting an employee to work honestly need not be stated; it is implied in the contractual relationship between employer and employee.

If a legally binding contract is made and one party to the contract breaches it, that party can be sued by the other for damages or for some form of restitution that would compensate the party against whom the breach was made for any losses that would have been incurred by the breach. In contract law, when one party is made to compensate another party it is not for punitive reasons, but to make sure that nobody is left in a worse position than they were before entering into the contract.

CONTRACTS IN PRACTICE

A practitioner who sees public patients will enter into a contractual relationship with the NHS. The contract is one in which the practitioner offers to deliver sight-testing services in return for payment from the NHS. For optometrists, the terms of service are stipulated in the regulations for provision of General Ophthalmic Services (Schedule 1, Regulation 2(1), national Health Service (GOS) Regulations 1986). These terms describe the premises where services can be provided, the requirements for adequacy of space and suitability of equipment, identify notices that must be displayed and indicate the minimum period for record retention. These terms oblige contracted practitioners to report any convictions or police cautions that they may have, stipulate who a practitioner can employ to test sight and who may deputize for them, require establishment of a complaints procedure in the practice, specify how payment is to be made and the duties required when testing sight. The Regulations also specify the details that the practitioner must provide and undertakings that he or she must make in order to be permitted to provide General Ophthalmic Services and list the groups of patients eligible to avail themselves of these services. (In Scotland, the contract for eye care provision extends beyond the GOS Regulations to incorporate a health assessment rather than primarily providing a sight test – Section 13, Smoking, Health and Social Care (Scotland) Act 2005.)

If a practitioner does not abide by the terms of the contract with the NHS, the health authority is permitted to:

- withhold payment if there has been a breach of terms of service;
- investigate whether the issuing of optical vouchers has been excessive;
- inspect premises and patients' records (giving the practitioner at least 14 days' notice).

In addition to a contract with NHS, practitioners may have individual contracts with suppliers of instruments, frames, spectacles, contact lenses, with a landlord (if premises are being rented) and employment contracts with employees. In all cases the basic premise of an offer and acceptance, and the fundamental features that make the contract legal, will apply.

SUMMARY

Business can be an important part of healthcare practice and, although it is concerned with making a profit, this does not have to and should never undermine ethical practice. Contractual obligations that underlie business and healthcare practice are created by the formation of contracts. In order to be legally binding, a contract requires an offer, acceptance, validity, consideration and intention.

References

Beu D S, Buckley R, Harvey M G 2003 Ethical decision-making: a multi-dimensional construct. Business Ethics: A European Review 12(1): 88–107

Block W, Cwik P F 2007 Teaching business ethics: a 'classificationist' approach. Business Ethics: A European Review 16(2):98–106

Carlill v Carbolic Smoke Ball Company [1893] EWCA Civ 1, [1893] 1 QB 256. British and Irish Legal Information Institute. Online. Available: http://www.bailii.org/

Fitzgerald L, Ferlie E 2000 Professionals: back to the future? Human Relations 53(5):713–719

Friedman M 1970 A Friedman doctrine: the social responsibility of business is to increase its profits. New York Times Magazine, September 13:32–33, 122–126

Griffin G R 1991 Machiavelli on management: playing and winning the corporate power game. Praeger, New York

Hafferty F 1988 Theories at the crossroads: a discussion of evolving views of medicine as a profession. Millbank Quarterly 66(2):202–205

Klempner G 2006 Ethics and advertising. In: Gunning J, Holm S (eds) Ethics, law and society, vol. 2. Ashgate Publishing, London, pp 219–224

Mason E S, Mudrack P E 1997 Are individuals who agree that corporate social responsibility is a fundamentally subversive doctrine inherently unethical? Applied Psychology: An International Review 46:135–152

Mudrack P 2007 Individual personality factors that affect normative beliefs about the rightness of corporate social responsibility. Business and Society 46(1):33–62

National Health Service (General Ophthalmic Services) Regulations 1986 Online. Available: http://www.assoc-optometrists.org/uploaded_files/consolidated_gos_regulations_1986.pdf

Smoking, Health and Social Care (Scotland) Bill 2005 Online. Available: http://www.opsi.gov.uk/legislation/scotland/acts2005/20050013.htm

Vogel D 1991 The ethical roots of business ethics. Business Ethics Quarterly 1(1):101–120

11

Ethical dilemmas

A dilemma is a situation in which it is difficult to know what choice to make. The difficulty arises because, no matter what decision is made, the consequences of that decision will be problematic. An ethical dilemma presents a person with a conflict: choosing between two or more actions, all of which may be ethically justified, yet each of which may result in some harm. In other words, an act that may be conducted with good intentions may not result in entirely good consequences. Ethical dilemmas can occur when ethical principles conflict; for example, choosing to respect the autonomy of an overweight individual to continue to overeat has bad consequences for health and is contradictory to beneficence. They can also occur when there are moral and legal issues involved.

DILEMMAS FROM CASE LAW AND MEDICINE

Philosophers offer many different types of hypothetical dilemma that generally present extreme situations in order to challenge ethical principles and moral reasoning. Yet extreme and even highly improbable circumstances are not necessarily impossible. The following could easily have come from a philosophical case study and yet is a real, albeit bizarre, case in English law.

The sailors who ate the cabin boy

Following a shipwreck, four sailors were cast adrift without food and with no impeding rescue. Almost 3 weeks later the sailors were close to death from starvation. The youngest and slightest of the four, the cabin boy, was also the weakest and allegedly the closest to death. Two of the sailors killed and ate him. They were eventually rescued and tried for murder. In their defence, they said that the cabin boy would have died from starvation anyway and, if they had not eaten him, they would also have died. Although this defence was not accepted, they were spared the death sentence, which was the punishment for murder, and given 6 months of hard labour. (From the case of R v Dudley and Stephens [1884].)

Killing a person is wrong. It is wrong in law, it is unethical, and it is immoral. Yet some people would argue that this could not be a universally applied statement because it makes no mention of the situation or of the condition of the killer and victim. The above illustrates an extreme situation in which the choice meant abiding by the principle that killing is wrong and all sailors dying from starvation, or deciding that the death of one may save the others. This meant deciding which life was most worthy of being saved and hence which should be sacrificed. It may well have been the case that the cabin boy was closest to dying, but this could not be proved. The alternative reasoning would be that, as he was the youngest, he may have had, potentially, the most years left to live and so was the one who ought to have been saved.

Extreme circumstances when choices involving life and death need to be made, and need to be made very quickly, test moral reason and ethical principles. Although few people, if any, in the developed world will ever find that they are so close to starvation and death that they consider eating another human being, death by starvation is all too common in the developing world. Yet, we do not hear of rampant cannibalism occurring in these places. Could this be because those who have so little food and who endure so much suffering have fewer demands than do the well fed (and sometimes overfed) citizens of the developed world? Actions can be guided by expectations and demands set by the lifestyle to which a person has become accustomed, but to what extent is the development of ethical principles influenced by expectations, life adaptations and habit? This is a question that cannot be answered simply. Indeed, it may not need an answer until a person's ethical principles are challenged by a dilemma. Only then can some perspective on the limits of adhering to personal ethical principles become evident.

Starvation may be rare in the developed world, but decisions about life and death still need to be made. As new treatments are discovered, the lives of people who have suffered from terrible trauma or who suffer from a chronic illness can be saved. The case of the conjoined twins, Jodie and Mary (mentioned in Chapter 1), illustrates, in many respects, a similar dilemma to that of the sailors and the cabin boy: the choice is between unquestioningly respecting the sanctity of life (even though it is a life close to death) or taking that life to save another. In some cases the patient does not wish to be saved, either because a chronic disease is too painful or because they would be left to live with disability and incapacitation. In such situations, doctors and, sometimes, family members are confronted with the dilemma of saving a life against the wishes of the patient.

The story of Dax

Donald (Dax) Cowart was a young man in his mid-twenties when he was severely injured in an accident that claimed his father's life. He suffered horrific burns over 65% of his body. He also lost his sight, and his ears and hands were badly damaged. He begged to be allowed to die rather than to have to undergo the daily rituals of excruciatingly painful but life-saving treatment. The doctors at the hospital, however, sought consent from his mother to continue treatment even though she was not a legally appointed guardian and Dax was an autonomous adult who, after psychiatric evaluation, was deemed to be fully capable of making his own decisions. His mother wanted the doctors to do all they could to save her son's life.

The doctors faced a dilemma: whether to take into account the wishes of the mother and try to save the patient's life, or to respect the choice and autonomy of the patient. They chose the former course of action and Dax's life was eventually saved, even though he was left disfigured. He attempted suicide twice after rehabilitation. In time he went on to complete a law degree and he married. The settlement from the oil company, whose negligence led to the accident, secured his future financially. Yet, Dax still maintains that his autonomy should have been respected. (Cowart 1988, 1994)

This case has been seminal in progressing respect for patient autonomy in the United States.

The dilemma in the case of Dax Cowart was a very poignant and complex one between preserving life and respecting autonomy. Doctors have a duty to save and protect life, and this is considered to be beneficent. In circumstances where the patient is in a vegetative state and is kept alive by artificial means, the courts have allowed the life support machines to be turned off (Airedale NHS Trust v Bland [1993]). Dax, however, was not dependent on life support but he certainly would have died if his wounds had been left untreated. An autonomous adult has the choice of refusing or accepting treatment, and that choice should be respected. Dax was an autonomous adult but the doctors considered his choice so extreme that they turned to his mother to make decisions for him. The underlying dilemma in this case was the one faced by Dax's mother. She was in an extremely difficult position of having to choose between abiding by her son's wishes or giving doctors permission to save his life, i.e. to respect her son's autonomy or to do what she considered to be beneficent. A mother will normally do all she can to protect and save the life of her child, so it was not surprising that Dax's mother asked the doctors to do all that was possible to save his life. However, by so doing, she was compelling Dax to undergo extremely painful treatments and ultimately to live with disfigurement and disability, something that at that time he did not want. It is debatable whether the choice that Dax's mother made was, indeed, beneficent from the point of view of the patient.

EMPATHY IN DECISION-MAKING

Making a decision for another person requires a great deal of empathy with that person and effort taken to understand their situation and how they may feel about it. Beneficence, from the perspective of the patient, should be considered. Such a decision will always be more complicated if it is confounded by emotion: the love of a parent for a child, the love of a child for a parent, the love of a man or woman for a partner.

In the clinical setting, emotion generally does not and should not, if possible, confound decisions. If a patient looks to a clinician for a decision, the clinician should assess the options and choose the course of action that gives the best possible outcome. If a dilemma arises, empathy with the patient may help to make the decision, but this should be balanced against clinical, medical and scientific knowledge.

Clinical case study

A 34-year-old patient comes in for a routine examination. Ophthalmoscopy reveals a large pigmentation on the retina, the shape of which resembles a malignant tumour. The patient is referred to a specialist and returns the following week in tears. The specialist has confirmed that the pigmentation is a malignant growth that is spreading rapidly, and has told the patient that the only way to prevent the cancer spreading is to enucleate the eye. The patient says that she cannot face this and would rather die than have an eye removed. She says that she will seek other ways that this tumour could be treated and cured. When you say that there is no other treatment of which you are aware that can treat or cure the cancer and that enucleation is the only way to save her life, she asks your opinion about a complementary therapy that she has heard cures cancer. It is offered in Switzerland and there is a 12-month waiting list for treatment.

You have heard about this treatment and that, whilst not every patient who has undergone the treatment has had a regression of cancer, the therapy has no known side-effects. You explain to the patient that, by waiting for such a long period, the tumour may spread so far that it could be fatal. The patient tells you that the waiting time can be reduced considerably, to a few weeks, if she has a supporting or referring letter written by a primary care practitioner such as you. She begs you to help her.

Would you comply with the wish of the patient and write a letter of referral to the Swiss therapy clinic, or would you try to convince her to undertake the orthodox treatment?

In some ways this case is similar to that of Dax Cowart. Treatment is offered to save a patient's life but it will result in loss of a part of the body. Like Dax, the patient in the case study is opposed to the treatment. She is adamant that she does not want to lose her eye. Her situation is perhaps less immediately serious and far less painful than the situation that Dax faced: she will not be left blind or disfigured. She wants to continue living with two healthy eyes and will do anything to preserve this situation. She rejects the orthodox treatment and cannot be forced to undergo it. In this case the autonomy of the patient and her right to choose should be respected.

The additional factor to consider is that this patient is requesting the practitioner's help in an action that, although not conventional, may not necessarily be wrong and may even offer a better outcome than can be provided by the orthodox treatment. Complementary therapies are more accepted in certain European countries, and many people use them in preference to orthodox medicine. Whilst there is no certainty that the treatment will work, there is no clear evidence that it will not work. If there is even the remotest possibility that it will be successful, should the patient not be given every chance to try it? This has to be balanced against the risk involved in delaying orthodox treatment by a few weeks. This may be a dilemma between respect for autonomy and beneficence/non-maleficence, but that depends on how beneficence and non-maleficence are judged. From the perspective of the patient it would be more beneficent to try the complementary therapy and, if this does provide a remedy, it would surely be the most non-maleficent compared to enucleation.

Yet, some practitioners may not judge the beneficence and non-maleficence of an action and outcome in the same way as the patient. In this case, a practitioner may be concerned about supporting the patient in trying a complementary therapy because such support may be considered as stepping beyond orthodox practice. The practitioner may fear being reported and suffering a slight to reputation. Whilst this is an understandable reaction, the fear of losing reputation should be balanced against what is best for the patient. Is it more important to respect the wishes of the patient and to do whatever is possible to save the eye, or should preservation of professional standing have the greater priority? It may help if the practitioner puts him or herself in the position of the patient. Would the practitioner risk delaying orthodox treatment for a few weeks to try something unknown that may have the potential to save their eye? The decision, in such a case, will depend on how much trust the practitioner has in unconventional or complementary therapies as well as how much emphasis he or she places on patient views and opinions. A practitioner who considers that it is their role to guide and control the decision-making process is less likely to follow the wishes of the patient than one who feels, particularly in such a case as this, that patient choice is paramount.

DILEMMAS ARISING BECAUSE OF CONFLICTS BETWEEN ETHICAL PRINCIPLES

Each of the ethical principles described in previous chapters can, in certain situations, conflict with one or more of the other principles, and following one principle requires going against another. When this arises in clinical practice, practitioners need to be able to justify to themselves why they followed a particular course of action rather than a different course. Whilst practitioners try to do what is best for the patient and to minimize or avoid causing the patient harm, there are times when it is not clear what is best. Certain clinical treatments may be both beneficial and harmful, and assessing the risks and benefits may show that both are relatively high. A good example of this is the use of orthokeratology on young children in order to prevent progression of myopia. Orthokeratology is not without risks of infection and damage to sight, and these risks may be higher in children (Young et al 2004). Yet, there is evidence that orthokeratology may retard the progression of myopia (Cho et al 2005). The dilemma in this case is between beneficence and non-maleficence: a balance between doing the best to treat the myopia and trying to avoid causing harm. The risks and the potential benefits of orthokeratology exceed any possible risks and benefits of the common alternative to treating myopia: prescribing spectacles. The practitioner needs to decide whether or not he or she is prepared to accept higher risks for potentially greater benefits. In many cases the patient may request the treatment, and the principle of respect for autonomy also needs to considered.

Some of the most difficult dilemmas between ethical principles arise where patient lifestyle choices have and are damaging their health. Examples of this are smoking and over-eating – common causes of illness that can be fatal, yet no practitioner can take extreme measures, in the interests of beneficence, to force a patient to stop indulging in these habits. Autonomy will always have precedence in such cases because smoking and excessive eating are not illegal activities. Society requires that we respect the choices of other people, provided these choices are not harming others and are not against the law. To stop people harming themselves requires laws that forbid harmful behaviour. In the case of smoking, measures to curb and restrict the habit have been introduced, but they do not make smoking illegal *per se*, they merely legislate where smoking is not permitted. Patients retain the choice of whether to smoke or not.

Should the behaviour of the patient be taken into account when trying to determine the best course of action? When resources are limited, it could be argued that justice demands that patients who are ill through no fault of their own should be given preference before those who have contributed to their own illness. This argument can be difficult to sustain when a choice has to be made between giving preferential treatment to a very elderly woman who

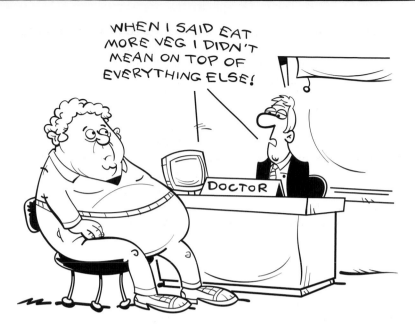

is ill through no fault of her own or giving the treatment to a single mother of three young children who has a chronic condition because of poor lifestyle choices. The elderly woman may be considered the more deserving, if patient behaviour is taken into account. However, denying help to the single mother could deprive three young children of vital care. The ethical dilemma between choosing what is just (being most fair to the most deserving patient) and what is beneficent (doing the most good) sometimes needs to take into account the personal situation of the patients and how the choice of action may affect others. In the case of whether to treat the elderly woman or the single mother, the outcome of the chosen action on the children should also be considered.

DILEMMAS ARISING BECAUSE OF CONFLICT BETWEEN ETHICS AND MORALITY

Amongst the most controversial topics in medical ethics are those in which basic moral principles are evoked; these can sometimes involve a perceived challenge to religious beliefs and practices. Abortion is one such issue that continues to provoke heated debate. The arguments centre on the opposing rights of the mother and those of the unborn child, and the differences of opinion about what constitutes a human being and the point at which life begins. These differences have become further confounded with the progress in technology and the ability of doctors to save the life of some prematurely born children at 22 weeks' gestation. Abortion can be permitted up to 24 weeks of pregnancy in England, Scotland and Wales (this does not apply to Northern Ireland where abortion can be only carried out on strictly medical grounds). This introduces a dilemma: if the life of a child can be considered worth saving at 22 weeks' post-conception because it is born prematurely, can it be right to abort an unborn fetus at 22, 23 or 24 weeks of gestation?

The ethical issues are underpinned by moral views about sexual relations and the responsibility for their consequences. Religious groups opposed to abortion point to the consequences on morality of making abortion available on demand. Some doctors refuse to perform abortions because they are opposed on religious and/or moral grounds to the procedure.

There are many other instances where the moral views of a practitioner can influence ethical principles and choices of action. An area in which this can occur is cosmetic surgery when it is performed to enhance appearance. There is no doubt that this is a lucrative area. Payment comes from wealthy patients and not from the public purse. The controversy is whether or not it is ethical to perform a surgical procedure and therefore put the patient at risk when there is no illness or condition that requires treatment or a cure. The added moral dimension is whether it is acceptable for practitioners to be indulging the vanities of the rich and making a financial gain from such practice when surgical skills and expertise are needed to help those who need life-saving operations. Cosmetic surgery would certainly appear to violate the Hippocratic Oath. The arguments in support of cosmetic surgery are that practitioners are helping people who wish to improve their appearance as this may have a positive effect on their well-being and confidence, and that how a person earns and spends their money, as long as it is legal, should be a matter of personal choice.

In eye care, laser surgery for correcting refractive error has parallels to cosmetic surgery. It is not essential for improving health and is often chosen to improve appearance by removing the need for spectacle correction. Whilst the issue of whether or not laser eye surgery is a purely cosmetic procedure remains contentious, similar ethical and moral arguments to those used for and against cosmetic surgery could be applied.

It is notable that, as with the pro-abortion advocates, those who support cosmetic surgery for improvement of appearance do not rely on morality to advance their case; the issues are more likely to be grounded on support for autonomy and the right of the patient to make a choice. When the ethical dilemma, as cited here, involves issues of morality, the dilemma is often one of an ethical principle pitted against a moral belief.

DILEMMAS ARISING BETWEEN ETHICS AND THE LAW

In a society regulated by laws, in most situations and for most people there is no question of a choice in a course of action when the choices are between an action that is lawful and one that involves breaking the law. Yet, instances can arise when law-abiding individuals may choose to break the law for reasons they feel that they can justify, for example, a man who exceeds the speed limit because his wife has just gone into labour in the car. For the husband in this particular situation, following the law would appear to provide a worse outcome than breaking it. Laws are set for the good of all, or at least for the greater good, and there will always be laws and regulations that some members of society find unjust or wrong, or perhaps restrictive in certain circumstances. Yet, clearly, laws cannot be written to cater for individual wants, needs or circumstances: bespoke laws would not be workable. Situations can arise in which following the law may not appear to be the fairest thing to do.

The butler's dilemma

A butler works in the service of a reclusive billionaire. One morning he goes into the bed chamber to wake the billionaire and finds that he has died in his sleep. Amongst the billionaire's many valuable possessions there is a large piece of jewellery about which nobody but the butler knows. The butler could take this piece of jewellery, sell it, and send the proceeds to a charity that works to alleviate poverty in Africa. The value of the

Continued

jewellery is such that money obtained by its sale could provide sufficient food for an entire village for a year. If the jewellery is left where it is, a very wealthy member of the billionaire's family will eventually claim it. *(Based on The Butler's Dilemma by Scott Adams)*

Should the butler take the jewellery and use it to benefit those who are in need, or should he leave it?

Taking the jewellery would amount to theft. The fact that the butler would never be caught and that his intentions may be noble does not take away from the fact that this would be a crime. There are those who would argue that the distribution of wealth in the world is so grossly unjust that the law should not protect the very wealthy to the extent that it does, and should not prevent any attempts to more fairly redistribute their riches. Those who support this argument would say that the butler is taking the jewellery not for personal gain but to help others. The billionaire is now dead, so has no use for the valuable, and his relatives, who are sufficiently rich, are unaware of its existence. Hence, by taking the item, nobody would suffer any loss and a whole village would benefit. This is a Robin Hood approach to justice: to take from the rich and give to the poor.

Those who favour this means of spreading justice often point to the way that wealthy nations exploit and mistreat the poor and developing countries, and that morally, if not legally, this exploitation is a form of crime. It is indisputable that the distribution of wealth in the world is unjust and disproportionate and that there is a reluctance to redress this, particularly amongst some of the wealthiest individuals in the world. However, to take forcibly and without legal basis from the rich, or to do so without their knowledge, to give to the poor undermines a basic principle in our law: to respect others and their possessions. There are legal and political ways of securing fairer wealth distribution (e.g. higher taxes for the wealthy) and sharing global resources. To operate outside the law is to disrespect the organization of society, and if this were promulgated on a larger scale it would lead to social disorder and chaos. The protection that the laws give to people would be eroded and this would ultimately work against the greater good and could lead to greater injustice.

There are situations in which an obligation to the law may not be quite as clear.

Clinical case study

A young man presents to your practice late on a Friday afternoon. You have never seen him before and he says that he has recently moved to the area. He complains about a severe itching in one eye and you see that the eye is red. The receptionist and all other staff have left. You have some time and agree to see the patient. The irritation is minor and turns out to have been caused by a contact lens that has been put in the wrong way around. After the examination the patient thanks you and leaves. He is particularly grateful to you for accepting him at short notice, because he tells you that he is leaving for an overseas holiday in a few days and did not want to be burdened with an ocular irritation.

The following Wednesday you sit down to the evening news and you hear that the police are looking for a young man suspected of plotting terrorist activity. The face that is shown on television bears a resemblance to the young man who presented at your practice the previous week with a red eye. The police say that they have been following him for some time and there was a reported sighting of him on Monday. As his identity is known to the Home Office and had been forwarded to all airports he could not have left the United Kingdom, and the police suspect that he is hiding somewhere close to home. The town cited is some 100 miles from your practice. The name that is stated on the news is not the same as the name that the patient gave to you. The police ask for anyone who may have had contact with the suspect to report this.

You are not entirely certain that the patient you saw is the same person as the suspect, although there is a distinct resemblance.

Would you provide the details of this patient to the police because, although you are not entirely sure about whether your patient and the suspect are one and the same, you may be instrumental in averting a serious attack on the public? Or would you consider that, as you are not completely sure that this is the same person, it is not worth the risk of breaching confidentiality and putting a potentially innocent person under suspicion? The police have not approached you, so you are not under any legal obligation to provide personal data.

This is a dilemma that involves choosing to protect the confidentiality of a patient or deciding that this may be a legal matter and that breaching confidentiality would be in the interests of the public. The decision may depend on how the practitioner feels about civil liberties and national security. Reporting the patient may result in an innocent man being detained and deprived of his liberty. Although not common, innocent people have been falsely accused of crimes and erroneously charged. Charging an innocent person leaves the true perpetrator at large. The opposing argument would be that it is better to be safe, even if that means subjecting an innocent person to police checks and possible short-term detention for, if the patient is not the suspect, the police should discover this and release him. This argument relies on complete trust in the competence of the police and criminal justice system. A choice such as this needs to be considered very carefully as the repercussions are serious: reporting the patient could potentially destroy the reputation and life of another person; not reporting could be instrumental in leading to large-scale death and destruction.

Sometimes a dilemma can occur between ethics and practice rules/regulations. When treating patients, there may be instances in which a practitioner wants to devote more time and perhaps more resources to a certain patient and this may conflict with rules established in the practice. An elderly woman suffers a heart attack in the examination room and the practitioner and receptionist are the only staff members at the practice. The practitioner wants to stay with the patient until the ambulance arrives, but this will impinge on the consultation time given to the next patient who has travelled a long distance for the examination and may have a limited amount of time in which to wait. Should the practitioner adhere to the rules of the practice, giving the allocated time to each patient, or can these rules by bent or broken in an extreme situation? The practitioner has to decide where the greater need lies and what action will provide the best outcome: to stay with the first patient or to leave the receptionist with this patient until the ambulance arrives and to devote the allotted time to the second patient. The situation would be made more difficult if the patient who had suffered the heart attack was the practitioner's mother. Deeper emotions would surely be stirred and these may affect judgement and the choice of action.

Of course, practice rules are not laws and therefore the consequences of bending these and making adjustments in extreme circumstances or in an emergency will not incur a legal penalty. In this hypothetical case, the patient who has travelled a distance for an examination may be understanding of the situation and prepared to reschedule the appointment. How a practitioner behaves in such a circumstance depends on how much they believe in adherence to rules and how extreme they consider that circumstances should be before a rule can be bent or broken.

SUMMARY

The choice that a practitioner makes when faced with a dilemma will depend on a number of factors: personal beliefs and morals, how the practitioner assesses and rates risk and benefits, and how far he or she is prepared to agree with patient choice even when this is contrary to what the practitioner may think or know is best. As long as the practitioner has the best interests of the patient at heart and is able to justify the chosen course of action, the decision ought not to be deemed unethical.

References

Adams S 2007 The butler's dilemma. Online. Available: http://dilbert-blog.typepad.com/the_dilbert_blog/2007/04/the_butlers_dil.html

Airedale NHS Trust v Bland [1993] AC 789, 805

Cho P, Cheung S W, Edwards M 2005 The longitudinal orthokeratology research in children (LORIC) in Hong Kong: a pilot study on refractive changes and myopia control. Current Eye Research 30:71–80

Cowart D 1988 Patient autonomy: one man's story. Journal of the Arkansas Medical Society 85(4):165–169

Cowart D 1994 An interview with Dax Cowart. Interview by Eric A Rosenberg and Demetrios A Karides. Journal of the American Medical Association 272(9):744–745

R v Dudley and Stephens [1884] 14 QBD 273

Young A L, Leung A T S, Cheng L L, Law R W K, Wong A K K, Lam D S C 2004 Orthokeratology lens-related corneal ulcers in children: a case series. Ophthalmology 111:590–595

Philosophy and ethical theory

THE PRACTICE OF ETHICS

Human behaviour, the way people treat one another, the choices and actions that different individuals make and the reasons that are given for making such choices are all fundamental themes in ethical theory and topics in applied ethics. The explanations of ethical behaviour and moral reasoning are firmly grounded in the realm of philosophy. The various schools of philosophical thought offer a diverse range of approaches and perspectives to the study and understanding of ethics.

In order to understand and distinguish between the different philosophical approaches it is best to look at their broad classifications and subclassifications. Bowie (2004) has expressed the three ways of practising ethics as:

- *Normative/traditional* – looking at behaviour that is right and wrong, at moral choices that should be made and at the application of appropriate rules
- *Descriptive/comparative* – comparing different approaches to behaviour and morality in different societies
- *Meta-ethics* – studying the actual meaning and function of words such as 'right' and 'wrong'.

Within each of these practices, there are further layers of subclassification. To delve into each is beyond the scope of this book. With respect to health care, the theories of normative ethics have the greatest application.

WHAT IS MORE IMPORTANT: THE MEANS OR THE ENDS?

The ethical choices that an individual makes and the moral reasoning behind these choices lead to actions and these actions have consequences. A common philosophical debate in normative ethics is whether the moral reasoning and the ethical choice should be based on the morality of the action or on the benefit brought about by the consequences of the action. Broadly speaking, normative ethics can be subdivided into theories that are concerned with actions (deontological) and those that are concerned with the consequences of actions (teleological).

Deontology and duty-based ethics

"So act, that the rule on which thou actest would admit of being adopted as a law by all rational beings."

Immanuel Kant in the *Metaphysics of Ethics*

Deontology, derived from *deon*, the classical Greek word for duty, considers the morality of actions rather than their consequences. This theory maintains that duty and the action involved in doing this duty and following a set of rules is of paramount importance. In other words, individuals should act in ways that are right and just even if the consequences of such behaviour do not always produce the maximum good.

The famous philosopher Immanuel Kant (1724–1804) was a proponent of this theory. Kant's philosophy was that a set of moral rules should be universally accepted not because they are imposed on people but because, if everyone followed these moral rules freely, they would become universal. Society would then be made up of autonomous individuals who chose to follow the same moral rules and could coexist in harmony, respecting the autonomy of others. This philosophy links morals to free will and to respect for autonomy. It stipulates that actions should follow laws and moral rules for no other reason than that it is right to do so. If the action does also happen to bring about good consequences, that is a bonus, but the consequence should not be the reason for the action. In other words, people should do the right thing not because it will bring them or others benefits but simply because the action itself is right in accordance with a universal set of laws and morals (Kant 1785, as translated by Ellington 1983).

In support of deontology, this philosophy offers a fixed set of morals for determining choice of action and, if it could be willingly adopted in a society, it would offer a stable and harmonious environment. The difficulty with this theory is that it maintains that actions are either right or wrong. There is no flexibility to allow for different circumstances. It has also been argued by many opponents of deontology that an absolute set of moral principles does not exist and that an ultimate standard against which such a set would be measured has never been defined (Mill 1861). Therefore, say opponents, morality and ethical behaviour could never be determined by a universal and rigid set of principles.

Teleology and utilitarianism – the consequences of behaviour

"All action is for the sake of some end."

John Stuart Mill in *Utilitarianism*

Utilitarianism places greater prominence on the consequences of actions and asserts that individuals choose to behave in certain ways because they consider the effect of their actions on themselves and on others and make their choices based on consideration of the consequences. According to utilitarianism, an action is right if it leads to the greatest happiness; one that leads to unhappiness is wrong (Mill 1861). The notion of happiness as the underlying reason for action does not mean that behaviour should be determined purely by pleasure. This would be hedonistic and selfish. The happiness of which Mill and other utilitarian philosophers, such as Bentham (1789), speak is happiness for the individual as well as for the greatest number of people. Utilitarianism advocates consequences that can spread happiness and reduce or prevent unhappiness.

Happiness can be attained by striving for contentment, satisfaction and enjoying what life brings as well as by maintaining a general interest in the public good (Mill 1861). This would seem to be reasonable until one tries to apply it to the many people who lead unhappy lives through no fault of their own: they may be destitute or suffering from debilitating illness. Although these people may have reached a level of acceptance and even tolerance of their life, it would be unreasonable to expect them to be satisfied, joyful or concerned with public good. Utilitarianism answers this by advocating that the more fortunate should try to help those who are less so in order to help minimize their unhappiness and bring them some measure of happiness. Indeed, it has been argued that, as most of the unhappiness and evil in the world can be alleviated by the actions of society and individuals, those who are more fortunate are morally obliged to try to make the world a happier place (Mill 1861).

In contrast to deontology, the utilitarian approach would seem to be more flexible, because it does not specify that certain actions must be followed in order to behave ethically, but reasons that a number of different means may be used to reach the most beneficial end. The difficulty with this philosophy is that very few individuals are so completely selfless and so content with their own lives that they consider the good of all and act in accordance with this. It is not uncommon to find people in our society who obey the rule of law, work honestly, behave with integrity, and are kind and loving to their families and friends. Yet, when it comes to giving away some of their wealth to alleviate poverty and suffering in the world, they are reluctant to do so. They may even be disinclined to be charitable to the homeless in their society and on the streets of the cities where they live. These are decent law-abiding people, but they are not selfless. Their choices do not support the utilitarian view of moral behaviour. As such people are generally concerned about not breaking the law, if the government were to impose new laws requiring an extra income-based tax to be paid specifically to aid the homeless and impoverished, these people, who would otherwise avoid helping the less fortunate, would pay this tax. They would do so, not because they believe in utilitarianism and wish to spread happiness and make the world a better place, but because they adhere to the duties that the law imposes on them. This may appear to be a deontological approach to doing the right thing. Yet, it is not deontology in the strict sense because it is not a moral principle but an imposed law that is being followed.

ETHICAL THEORIES AND NATURAL JUSTICE

In contrast to ethics, when dealing with legal obligations there is generally less need for deciding a choice of action or for any deliberation about the consequences. If an individual does not wish to fall foul of the law, he or she will obey it. Deontology may be seen as somewhat closer to the law than utilitarianism in that deontology places a greater emphasis on duty and on doing the right thing according to a set of rules. Utilitarianism, however, may be perceived as more closely linked to natural justice and there is some recognition that people determine what is just depending on how well this promotes harmony and cohesion within a society (Mill 1861). Because the law is prescriptive there is a perception that the enforcement of law is at all times rigid and that, occasionally, this can be contrary to natural justice. Indeed, Kant perceived that practitioners of law (lawyers, judges) were always obliged to enforce it without question; the realm of querying and interpreting whether a law was fair belonged, according to Kant, to philosophers (Caygill 1995). Kant, were he alive today, might be surprised to discover that this is not quite true. Even within the relatively stringent rule of the law, flexibility can be introduced in cases where its absence could result in consequences that would be contrary to natural justice.

The law versus natural justice

A woman was brought before a magistrates' court for failing to pay council tax arrears of more than £2000. She stood in the dock expressionless and resigned. She had no legal representation and, after the council representative had presented the charges against her, she was asked by the magistrates for an explanation of why payment had not been made. Her answer was that she had no money left to pay the tax. Her income and outgoings were assessed and it was clear that she had less than £1 left each month in spite of the fact that she had cut all spending to bare essentials.

The woman was a single mother to a 9-year-old child. The father of the child had abandoned her years ago and had never helped with maintenance. She worked part-time doing domestic duties for minimal wages. She had

Continued

done this for 18 years and, because she had a job, however lowly paid, she did not qualify for any means of financial assistance. (In effect, had she chosen not to work, she would have been more secure financially and would have qualified for assistance with council tax payments). Given the amount of council tax in arrears and the inability to pay, the woman faced a 3-month prison sentence. The presiding magistrates decided that, in the interests of justice, all arrears should be remitted.

A case in which the author was one of the presiding magistrates.

Whilst it is generally accepted that all members of a society should be bound by the same laws and regulations, it could be argued that some of these laws, in certain situations, appear to be unjust to the poorer members of society. The law states that tax needs to be paid on earnings by everyone ... everyone except those who are exempt – and some of these exemptees are the richest people in the United Kingdom. Those who name their official residence as being outside the country (or whose earnings go to their overseas resident spouses) are entitled to benefit from great reductions in tax payment. Phillip Green, one of the richest men in England, was not required by law to pay tax on the billion pound bonus that he awarded himself because this was made out in the name of his wife, who is resident in Monaco. Whether these laws are just, or whether the billionaires and millionaires who take advantage of such laws are behaving morally and ethically, may be questionable, but it is nonetheless perfectly legal.

The imbalances that occur in society because of laws like these do result in vast wealth differences and some people find themselves destitute. It was because of such imbalances that a hard-working single mother found herself in front of a court facing a prison sentence. In such cases, the law can and, depending on the judge or magistrate, usually does try to make adjustments and amendments. This does not mean an abrogation of legal obligations: wilful refusal of council tax payment carries a prison sentence. It means that justice can and should prevail when strict enforcement of the law could inadvertently lead to injustice.

A duty-bound approach to law would have required that, as it is moral and right to follow the law, and it is right to punish those who do not follow the law, the woman should have been sent to prison. She should have put the duty to pay the council tax before all else, regardless of the consequences (going without food and clothing for herself and her child). A more utilitarian view would maintain that she should consider the consequences, and that feeding her child had to come before the duty to pay the tax.

NORMATIVE ETHICS IN HEALTH CARE

Ethics in healthcare practice contains a mixture of deontological and teleological approaches; which one of the two is used may depend on the circumstance or on the practitioner. In some cases, situations dictate that one ethical approach is preferable to the other. It is the duty of the practitioner to do his or her best for the patient (beneficence) and to minimize harm (non-maleficence).

If a patient, who intends to drive, needs a refractive correction and cannot wear contact lenses, the practitioner will prescribe spectacles and strongly recommend that the patient wear these when driving. The practitioner is acting out of duty: it is the right thing to do to prescribe the spectacles and to recommend that they be worn. It could be that the practitioner also considers the consequences of the patient not wearing a correction whilst driving, as much for the patient as for any member of the public who may come into contact with the patient. In this case, whether the practitioner follows the deontological approach and does what is right and dutiful, or takes the utilitarian approach and acts in accordance with what would bring about the most beneficial consequences and make the patient happy, amounts to the same choice of action. If the patient, however, is reluctant to wear the spectacles and would be unhappy doing so, the duty of the practitioner does not alter: the practitioner is still obliged to issue a prescription and give sound advice. The fact that the actions of the practitioner may not make the patient happy needs to be disregarded. Here the duty to prescribe and recommend the wearing of the correction must prevail; acting to make the patient happy would be unsafe, irresponsible, and could lead to much greater misery.

VIRTUE ETHICS

Deontology and utilitarianism have in common a focus on actions and moral principles, whether it is doing the right thing or considering what consequences are the best. A third school of thought argues that ethical behaviour should not be determined solely by actions and principles but should also take into account the character of an individual. In other words, it is less concerned with what a person does and more with what a person is: with their good qualities, their virtues. According to this philosophy, an act is good and right if it is done by a virtuous person.

One of the advocates of this philosophy was Aristotle (384–322 BC). Aristotle considered that people should live in accordance with reason and that reason should be used to improve character by developing virtues (Aristotle, c330 BC, translated by Thomson 1953). He proposed that there were 12 moral virtues: courage, temperance, generosity, magnificence, magnanimity, proper desire for small honours (ambition), patience, truthfulness, wittiness, friendliness, proneness to shame (modesty), and proper indignation. Each virtue was associated with two vices: one that represents a deficiency in that particular virtue and one that represents an excess of it. For example, the virtue of courage has two associated vices: cowardice (too little courage) and rashness (too much courage). A person of good character chooses the mean between the two vices, in other words the virtue.

Proponents of virtue ethics point out that adherence to a set of rules is not a satisfactory way of determining what is ethical and what is not, because no moral rule can have universal application. Possessing a virtuous character does not require reliance on a set of rules because virtuous individuals know how to make a judgement about the appropriate action to take in any particular circumstance. If everybody lived a life devoted to the development of these virtues, it is possible that all people would indeed do what is right and that the consequences of human actions would, for the most part, be good. However, whilst this philosophy does not require a set of rules, it does depend on agreement about a common set of virtues and, more importantly, presupposes that the virtuous person is infallible. It is unreasonable to expect anyone, even the most virtuous, not to have occasional lapses of good character and behaviour.

VIRTUE ETHICS IN HEALTH CARE

A healthcare practitioner, as indeed any professional, is widely regarded as a person of integrity and there is an expectation that he or she will be of such character and show such behaviour as is associated with virtue. A practitioner is expected to be honest, friendly, courteous, kind, trustworthy and patient. These traits do not include the skill or expertise of the practitioner. Although skills, expertise and the requisite level of knowledge are also expected, these can be demonstrated by the fact that the practitioner holds the correct qualifications. For many patients this is sufficient evidence that the practitioner possesses the necessary expertise and knowledge. Traits of character are not recorded on a degree certificate and cannot be measured or tested quantitatively. Patients judge these by the manner in which a practitioner deals with them and their condition or problem. If a practitioner does not treat patients with courtesy or is found to be dishonest, or is clearly more interested in the status and earnings that accompany the position and not with patient care, this will become evident to patients and to colleagues.

It is important, however, in healthcare practice, as indeed in any profession where one is helping people, that a clear distinction is made between the character of the practitioner and how this character may be perceived. Practitioners who appear to lack the qualities associated with good character may not necessarily be bad people or, indeed, incompetent practitioners. There may be instances when an apparent lack of care or goodwill towards patients is not caused by the practitioner lacking in 'virtue', but that the practitioner has mistakenly chosen the wrong profession. Not every person of virtue or good character is suited to healthcare practice. Whilst virtue should transcend the boundaries of activity and occupation (a good person is good regardless of what they do for a living), it can be difficult not to show frustration and mask good qualities when in a job one does not enjoy. Such a practitioner may eventually leave healthcare practice and find a more suitable profession. They should do so without feeling that they have failed or are lacking.

There may also be cases in which the practitioner is a highly skilful as well as a caring individual who genuinely enjoys healthcare practice, but who is not naturally inclined to instantaneous smiling, 'small talk' and superfluous conversation – all examples of what have become regarded by some (most unfortunately and erroneously) as markers of 'good communication'. Whilst some patients may indeed prefer the chatty, smiling practitioner who can easily intersperse trivial talk amongst clinical questioning, there are many other patients who do not. Differences in personalities amongst the ranks of practitioners (as indeed amongst patients) should be respected and competence not judged on how a practitioner communicates or how often he or she smiles. The current over-emphasis on teaching a certain prescribed type of communication skill in universities has led to confusion, good students labelled as bad communicators, and students learning to 'act the part' rather than 'be the part'. Newly graduated practitioners may justifiably be mystified about how to communicate 'properly' with patients. It is important to remember that contrived 'caring' is not ethical, because it is a form of dishonesty. Patients can, in general, see through a less competent but charming 'actor' and appreciate the genuinely caring practitioner. The best form of communication comes from someone who genuinely cares and wants to help. When the empathy is felt and conveyed, the words used are more than likely to be interpreted correctly.

Misinterpretations can never be ruled out entirely, even for the very best and caring practitioner. A patient may have extremely high expectations of a practitioner, make unreasonable demands or even harbour a particular prejudice. In such cases, if an attempt is made by the patient to undermine the credibility or good character of the practitioner, he or she should hold firm to their practice and methods. If the practitioner has behaved ethically towards the patient, it would be wrong to try to pretend otherwise and appease a patient who is behaving unfairly, as this implies that the practitioner was in error. In such circumstances, the practitioner should be able to rely on the support of colleagues.

SOCIETY AND ETHICS – PATERNALISM

Society needs laws to maintain order and to protect all members of that society from harm. In certain instances, the protective effect of the law is seen as the government directly or indirectly interfering with and restricting individual choice and action. This is paternalism: the government deciding, like a father, what is best for the people. A ban on smoking in public places is an example of a government edict restricting an activity in order to protect the health of the public. It could be argued that in countries where there is a democratically elected government, the people have chosen those who will make the laws and so it is with the agreement of the people that any restrictions are introduced.

Mill, in 1859, pointed out that the agreement or will of the people does not include the will of *all* people. The same can be said today: there is no elected government that has been given a mandate to govern by all the people over whom it governs. Some are excluded from the process of electing the government, some have excluded themselves by choosing not to vote and some will have voted for a different party and may find their views unrepresented. It would clearly be difficult, if not impossible, to exempt those who did not vote for a particular government from the laws that the government makes. So people broadly, although perhaps in some cases grudgingly, accept that laws should be obeyed, even though some may be opposed to the restrictions and to the government that introduced them.

Questions about paternalistic behaviour have been very prominent since the disaster of 11 September 2001 and the introduction of a spate of allegedly anti-terrorism laws that many believe to be an unnecessary erosion of civil liberties. All people who wish to travel by air have their bags and clothing thoroughly checked and X-rayed before they are allowed to board an aeroplane. The government and those who support these measures say that they are meant for the public good because they are designed to protect against terrorism. Opponents argue that these measures are excessive, innocent people are treated as potential suspects, whilst the extent of the threat and indeed the very people against whom we are to be protected are unknown.

There is, of course, a simple way to avoid being checked at airports, and that is not to travel by air. This is clearly not a useful suggestion if there are no alternative means of transportation, but where there is a choice any governmental impositions can be avoided. When it comes to health care, there are situations in which paternalism cannot be avoided.

PATERNALISM IN HEALTH CARE

When the government makes decisions about health care, they are made for the 'greater good'. Some limited choices do exist. Parents of very young children are strongly encouraged to have their children vaccinated with the three-part MMR vaccine in order to minimize the chance of an epidemic of mumps, measles or rubella. The decision whether or not vaccinate a child remains with the parents. In other cases the patient and their families have no choice and paternalism of the state is seen to interfere with respect for autonomy of the individual. Terminally ill patients who wish to die and to be assisted in this by relatives or friends are not permitted, in the

United Kingdom, to have treatment that would accelerate their death. This governmental stance has been attacked for being paternalistic and overprotective and continues to be a source of controversy.

Anti-drug legislation is another example of paternalism. The government makes these laws to prevent the widespread use of drugs (although it is debatable whether the measures taken have been effective) whilst opponents argue that, if illegal drugs were made legal, the burgeoning criminal fraternity behind the trafficking and supply would lose its reason to exist. Addicts could then be treated without fear of prosecution and those who wished to take drugs could continue to do so at their own peril. The problem with this approach is that it leaves the choice of whether or not to take up a very dangerous habit with individuals and some may be particularly vulnerable and require protection. The government sets out therefore to protect everyone by refusing to allow a choice (for those who wish to abide by the law).

Whilst there are some people who would like to see a relaxation of laws that they consider too restrictive of individual choice, others call on greater state intervention for lifestyle choices that can lead to illness. The rise in obesity, especially in young children, has frightening prospects and yet obesity can be prevented and it can be reversed. Obesity is not a disease but it has the potential to lead to serious and chronic illnesses that place an extra burden on healthcare resources. State intervention to restrict calorie intake and to prevent the consumption of fattening foods with little nutritional value could curb the rise in obesity and may even reverse the trend. The government could outlaw all fast foods and sugary drinks; it could monitor those who are overweight and tax them for excessive weight gain; greater fares could be charged on public transport for larger people. The list of state-imposed measures could go on, and may receive support from some quarters because of the potential for great benefits for the health of the nation. However, these measures would also receive great condemnation. Such a degree of state intervention would be considered unacceptable by many people as it appears to show a complete disregard for personal lifestyle choice and autonomy. The government does draw the line on excessive paternalism. It will act to protect people from dangerous habits that can be avoided (drugs, cigarettes) but not from excesses such as overeating that require a degree of self-discipline.

PROTECTING THE MOST VULNERABLE – CAN LOVE BE AN ASSAULT ON HUMAN RIGHTS?

Most emotive and controversial are cases that involve great tragedies and suffering, and in which the autonomy of the individual is seriously pitted against the protectionism of the state, doctors and/ or relatives. The case of Dax Cowart (described in Chapter 11) is one example of this. The case of Ashley X is another and raises some very sinister and frightening possibilities.

The case of Ashley X

Ashley (not her real name) was born with static encephalopathy that left her severely disabled and completely dependent on her parents. Ashley cannot walk, talk, or sit up. She is fed through a gastrostomy tube and has the developmental age of an infant. The prognosis her parents were given was bleak: no cognitive or neurological development was expected.

Just before reaching the age of six years, Ashley had started to show signs of pubic hair growth and within a year her breasts began to bud. Her parents were concerned that Ashley's growth would accelerate and that, as a result of this, she would be too heavy to lift, causing them problems in their ability to care for her in the future. The parents did not wish to have her institutionalized.

After extensive discussion and consultations with specialists, it was decided that it would be in Ashley's best interest to have her growth stunted and her physical development arrested. The specialists sought ethical approval for the treatment and it was granted. Ashley was injected with high levels of oestrogen to inhibit her bone growth and her breast buds were removed, as was her uterus – the latter procedure was undertaken to prevent the onset of menstruation. The major risk associated with taking high-dose oestrogen in adults is the development of thrombosis, especially in the deep veins; the risks for a child of so young an age are unknown.

A year after the operation, and whilst still taking estradiol on a daily basis, no complications had been reported (Gunther & Diekema 2006).

Ashley is a very young child and is severely disabled. She is not and never will be considered an autonomous adult. All decisions and choices will be made for her and she will not be able to say whether or not these are in her best interests or according to her wishes. Her total reliance on her parents leaves her completely vulnerable. Her parents are caring and loving but they made a choice to have Ashley's physical development arrested. This was done for reasons that many have considered acceptable, but many others have deplored. The fear amongst opponents of the 'Ashley treatment' is that it will set a precedent for treatment of other severely disabled children.

The ethics committee that approved the treatment noted that such cases should be considered on a case-by-case basis (Gunther & Diekema 2006) but if there are other similar cases approval may be easier to obtain. The ethical dilemmas posed by such cases and the philosophical debates that they provoke revolve around the rights of vulnerable individuals in society. The paternalistic interventions made on their behalf have been made possible by scientific, medical and technological advances; the laws to deal with the uncertain consequences that these advances offer lag far behind.

Whilst the government makes laws for the benefit of the people, it certainly does not do so out of love. Love, the greatest of all human feelings, can lead to the most protective measures and sometimes to the most controversial choices. The parents of Ashley, like the mother of Dax, made decisions for their child out of love and the understandable desire to protect her. Can protection based on love be taken too far?

Should we tell mother?

Two adult brothers faced a moral dilemma. Their elderly mother, who was in her nineties, had dementia and was resident in a nursing home. Although frail and suffering from memory lapses, there were times when she would suddenly remember one of her children, a relative, a friend or an incident. At these times, the communication between the elderly woman and her children was the most rewarding. The brothers had recently had to cope with the death of their sister. This had been fairly swift following a diagnosis of cancer. In the short time between the diagnosis and death, the sister had been too ill to visit her mother and the elderly woman had never mentioned her daughter.

The brothers agonized over whether or not to tell their mother that her daughter had died: to respect the fact that this is something a mother would want to know but at the risk of causing her great distress, or to let

Continued

her be at peace but ignorant of her daughter's death. In the end they decided not to tell their mother. They continue to live with the fear and anxi-
ety of their elderly mother one day remembering her daughter and asking
to see her. What will they tell her then?

*Based on a true story related to the author by Reverend Dr Johnston
McMaster, Irish School of Ecumenics, Trinity College, Dublin.*

The brothers had made a choice to protect their mother from grief and pain, but they questioned whether in so doing they had denied her knowledge of the truth about her daughter and the right that any parent has to grieve for her child.

FREEDOM OF THOUGHT– AN ETHICAL REQUIREMENT

In order to make ethical choices, a person needs to have a set of principles and morals that will form a basis for such decisions. These principles and morals need to be developed with deep reflection and challenged by life situations. Underlying this development of personal ethics is the essential requirement for freedom of thought. Much of what is currently shown on television and written in tabloid newspapers is not conducive to developing free, independent thought and an open-minded attitude. It is rather an attempt to create heroes and celebrities from people who lack the talents expected of celebrated people and in some cases are people whose ethics and morals are questionable, if at all existent.

The thinking individual, who has a well developed set of ethics and is prepared to stand up for their principles, may find life difficult and may be unpopular at times. It takes great courage, in the face of ridicule and threats, to do what Brian Haw did to show his opposition to the invasion and occupation of Iraq that many considered illegal. Millions of people were opposed to the invasion but only Brian was brave enough to forgo everything to stage a protest demonstration in London that has lasted for more than 6 years (in spite of the government taking legislative steps to have Brian moved). This is a form of ethics in action: standing up for one's principles. Throughout history, people like Brian Haw, and not the cult 'celebrities' created by the mass media, are the ones who have become heroes and examples for future generations. The ethical practitioner does not need to be a hero for millions, but an example of decency and integrity for patients and colleagues.

SUMMARY

Some ethical theories consider right and wrong actions; others take into account good character and virtues. Ethics and its applications in health care may involve all of these aspects. Above all, the development of a set of personal ethics requires the capacity for individual thought, the ability and will to reflect deeply, the power to question motives and behaviour of self and of others and the strength to make a stance to do what one believes to be right.

References

Aristotle *c*330 BC The Nicomachean ethics (trans. J A K Thomson J A K) Tredennick H (ed.) 1953 Penguin, London

Bentham J 1789 Introduction to the principles of morals and legislation. In: Warnock M (ed.) 1979 Utilitarianism, On Liberty, and Essay on Bentham, John Stuart Mill. Collins, Glasgow, pp 33–78

Bowie R 2004 Ethical studies, 2nd edn. Nelson Thornes, Cheltenham

Caygill H 1995 A Kant dictionary (referencing Kant I 1798 A conflict of the faculties). Blackwell, Oxford, p 271

Ellington J W (trans.) 1983 Immanuel Kant, Grounding for the metaphysics of morals, 1785. Hackett Publishing, Indianapolis, p 1–63

Gunther D F, Diekema D S 2006 Attenuating growth in children with profound developmental disability. Archives of Pediatric and Adolescent Medicine 160:1013–1017

Mill J S 1859 On liberty. In: Warnock M (ed.) 1979 Utilitarianism, On Liberty, and Essay on Bentham, John Stuart Mill. Collins, Glasgow, pp 126–251

Mill J S 1861 Utilitarianism. In: Warnock M (ed.) 1979 Utilitarianism, On Liberty, and Essay on Bentham, John Stuart Mill. Collins, Glasgow, pp 251–322

Index

A

abortion, ethical dilemmas, 181–182
accountability, 47
Adoption and Children Act 2002, 120
advertising, and business ethics, 167–169
age discrimination, 137
altruism, and medical profession, 21
American Optometric Association, Code of Ethics, 34
anti-drug legislation, and paternalism, 199
Antinori, Severino, 54, 55–56
AOP (Association of Optometrists), 157
Aristotle, 195
artificial ventilation, 177
Asclepius/Aesculapius (god of medicine and healing), 4, 5
Ashley X, case of, 200–201
assisted conception, ethical decisions, 55–56
Assisted Dying for the Terminally Ill Bill, 72
assisted suicide, 71, 72, 198–199
Association of Optometrists (AOP), 157
autonomy
    adults unable to exercise, 76–79
    best interests argument, 80–81
    case studies, 68, 70–71, 73, 80, 81

autonomy (Continued)
    children under 16, and Gillick competency, 74–76, 119
    consent or refusal of treatment, 177
        see also consent to treatment; refusal of treatment
    definitions, 65
    informing patients about risks, 68–69
    informing patients of condition and treatment options, 67
    limits of respect for, 71–72
    and morality, 189
    patient choices/decisions, 69–71
    principle, 67
    refusal of treatment, 73–74
    respect for, 65–83
    vulnerable patients, 81–83

B

bad news, disclosing, 14
behaviour, consequences of, 190–191
beneficence, 49–56
    see also good deeds, and ethical behaviour
    and autonomy, 70
    case study, 52–53
    compassion, 53–54
    forms of, 51–53
    and harm, 53–54

beneficence *(Continued)*
    prevention of, 62–63
    ideal, 51–52
    integral to clinical practice, 63
    judging of, 179
    and justice, 181
    life, protection of, 177
    limitations of, 50, 51
    and non-maleficence, 57
        see also non-maleficence
    obligatory, 51, 52
    patient desires, 54, 55–56
    refusal of treatment, 56
Bentham, Jeremy, 52, 190
best interests argument, patient
        autonomy, 80–81
BNP (British National Party), 37
Bolam test, breach of duty of care,
        145–146, 147
Bolitho test, breach of duty of care, 147
Book of the Soul *(Ruhnama)*, 9
British National Party (BNP), 37
bullying at work, employment law,
        138–139
business, essence of, 161–162
business ethics
    advertising, 167–169
    commerce or consultation, 163
    contract law, 169–172
    cosmetic surgery, 168
    Machiavellian techniques, 165, 166
    management ethics and social
        responsibility, 165–166
    manipulation, 168
    patient, customer distinguished,
        162–163
    patient choice, 163–165
    roots, 162
'but for' test, causation, 148–149

C

cancer, 73, 153, 178
cataracts, 74, 152–153
causation, breach of duty of care,
        148–151
character
    development of, 17
    traits, among professionals, 30, 196
    universal principles of, 16

charity, donating to, 50
children
    aged over 16, right to confidentiality,
        119
    aged under 16, and Gillick
        competency, 75, 119
    conjoined twins, ethical decisions,
        2–3, 176
    friends, choice of, 88
    obese, 82
    protecting, 109–112
    secrets, telling of, 104
    and sexual activity, 88
Christianity, 6, 85
Cicero, Marcus, 85
claim rights, 44
Climbié, Victoria, 110–112
Clinton, Bill and Roger, 11
College of Optometrists
        (United Kingdom)
    Code of Ethics and Guidelines for
        Professional Conduct, 34–35, 38
    on record retention, 157
    on vulnerable patients, 106
collegiality
    see also employment law
    altered behaviour, 127
    and business, 169
    case studies, 127–128, 130
    definition of 'colleague', 122–123
    duties of doctors to each other, 8
    erosion of, 127
    ethical codes, 6
    fellow practitioners, collegial
        relations with, 125–126
    generalizations and prejudice,
        124–125
    junior and senior optometrists,
        relationship between, 123
    problem recognition, 126–129
    respect and understanding,
        importance, 123
    socializing, 129
    support for colleagues, absolute or
        relative, 126
    threats to, 126–127
    unwelcome intervention, 130
comparative ethical practice, 188
compassion, 16, 53–54
competence, consent to treatment, 77

complementary therapies, vs. orthodox treatment, 179
confidentiality
  see also data protection; disclosures
  children, protecting, 109–112
    Gillick competency, and children under 16 years, 75, 119
  ethical codes, 38–39
  as ethical concept, 103–112
  in law, 113–121
  married couples, 119–120
  protecting the secret or the person, 105–112
  respect for as ethical obligation, 121
  self-harm or harm to others, preventing, 53–54, 56, 107–109
  vulnerable adult, protecting, 106–107
conjoined twins, ethical decisions, 2–3, 176
conjunctivitis, giant papillary, 56
consent to treatment
  autonomy, respect for, 177
  children under 16, 75
  ethical codes, 39
  and legal action, 36
  mental incompetence, 76–77
contact lenses
  advertising of, 168
  ethical decisions, 56
  myopia, correction, 58, 59
contact tonometry, 69, 152
continuous professional development requirement, 39
contract law, 169–171
  consideration requirement, 170, 171
  contracts in practice, 171–172
  intention requirement, 170, 171
  validity requirement, 170
conversion, religious, 12
co-operation, need for, 40
corneal damage/scarring, 60, 152
corneas, donation of, 3, 50
corrective justice, 95
cosmetic surgery, 168, 182, 183
Cowart, Donald (Dax), 176–177, 178, 200
CPD (continuous professional development requirement), 39
crime and punishment, legal justice, 86
customers, and patients, 162–163

D

damages claims, practitioner protection, 154
data protection
see also confidentiality; disclosures
  adverse reactions, reporting, 118
  case study, 117
  Data Protection Act 1998, 113, 114, 115, 116, 117, 157
  manual data, 116
  personal data, 113, 114–115, 118
  principles, 114
  record retention, 157
  referrals, 118
  relevant filing system, defined, 116
  sharing of data, 118
  types of data protected, 115
death of children, when justifiable, 2–3, 176
decisions, ethical
  see also dilemmas, ethical
  conjoined twins, separation, 2–3, 176
  empathy, in decision-making, 177–179
  in-vitro fertilization (IVF) treatment, 54, 55–56
  life and death choices, 175–176
  patients', respecting, 15, 69–71
  sight, threats to, 3–4
  vegetative states, and life support, 177
Declaration of Geneva (Physician's Oath) 1948, 7
deontology
  and duty-based ethics, 189–190
  healthcare practice, 194
  and law, 192
  utilitarianism contrasted, 191
  virtue ethics, 194
descriptive ethical practice, 188
diabetic retinopathy, and smoking, 51, 70
dignity, 45
dilemmas, ethical
  see also decisions, ethical
  abortion, 181–182
  AIDS patient, 3
  case law and medicine, 174–177
  conflicts between ethical principles, 179–181

dilemmas, ethical *(Continued)*
  cosmetic surgery, 182, 183
  empathy, in decision-making, 177–179
  ethics and law, 183–186
  ethics and morality, 181–183
  life and death decisions, 175–176
  practice rules/regulations, and ethics, 186
  sexual relations, 182
  vulnerable patients, protection, 201
disability discrimination, 87, 135–136
disclosures
  see also confidentiality; data protection
  permitted, 118–119
  requirement, legal, 39, 116–118
  Road Traffic Act 1988, 117
  unintended, 119–120
discrimination
  see also employment law
  age, 137
  case studies, 136
  direct, 132, 133, 137
  disability, 135–136
  fixed-term contracts, 137
  gender-based, 127–129, 132–133
  indirect, 132, 133–134, 137
  and justice, 87, 90
  part-time employment, 137
  permitting in healthcare practice, 134–135
  positive, 137
  and prejudice, 124
  protection against, 90
    specific grounds, 131–132
  Protection from Harassment Act 1997, 138
  racial *see* racial discrimination
  religious, 135
  sexual orientation, 136–137
  statutory provisions
    Disability Discrimination Act 1995, 135, 136
    Disability Equality (Sexual Orientation) Regulations 2003, 136
    Employment Equality (Age) Regulations 2006, 137
    Employment Equality (Age) Regulations (Northern Ireland) 2006, 137

discrimination *(Continued)*
    Employment Equality (Religion or Belief) Regulations 2003, 135
    Employment Equality (Sexual Orientation) Regulations (Northern Ireland) 2003, 136
    Fair Employment and Treatment (Northern Ireland) Order 1998, 135
    Fair Employment (Northern Ireland) Act 1989, 135
    Fixed-Term Employees (Prevention of Less Favourable Treatment) Regulations 2002, 137
    Part-time Workers (Prevention of Less Favourable Treatment) Regulations 2000, 137
    Race Relations Act 1976, 133–134
    Race Relations Act 1976 (Amendment) Regulations 2003, 134
    Race Relations Order (Amendment) Regulations (Northern Ireland) 2003, 134
    Racial and Religious Hatred Act 2006, 135
    Racial Relations (Northern Ireland) Order 1997, 133
    Sex Discrimination Act 1975, 132
    Sex Discrimination (Northern Ireland) Order 1976, 132
  victimization, 132–133, 134, 137
distributive justice *see* resource distribution
doctors, duties of, 7–8
Doctors of Optometry, qualification as, 33
Donoghue v Stevenson case, tort law, 142, 143–144
duties of doctors
  see also duty of care
  to each other, 8, 122
    see also collegiality
  in general, 7–8
  to patients, 8, 122
    see also patients
  performing to the best of abilities, 15
duty
  of care *see* duty of care
  and deontology, 192
  ethical behaviour, 1

duty *(Continued)*
  ethical concepts, 46
  law, duty-bound approach to,
    193–194
duty of care, 143–151
  breach of, 145–148, 159
    harm suffered from , 148–151
  neighbour principle, 144

E

effort and sacrifice, resource
    distribution, 97–98
elderly patients, communication with,
    77–78
empathy, in decision-making, 177–179
employment law, 130–139
  see also collegiality
  bullying at work, 138–139
  contracts of employment, 131
  discrimination *see* discrimination
  Employment Rights Act 1996, 131,
    138
  fast development of, 131
  Health and Safety at Work etc Act
    1974, 138
  master-servant relationship, 131
entertainment, recognition of, 27
enucleation treatment, cancer, 178
epilepsy, informing authorities about,
    108–109
equipment, old and malfunctioning,
    39–40
ethical codes, modern, 6–7
ethical concepts
  accountability, 47
  confidentiality as *see* confidentiality
  dignity, 45
  duty, 46
  principles, 45–46
  respect, 44–45
  responsibility, 46
  rights, 44
  standards, 46
  values, 43–44
  virtues, 43
ethical principles
  beneficence *see* beneficence
  collegiality *see* collegiality
  conflicts between, 15, 179–181

ethical principles *(Continued)*
  ethical concepts, 45–46
  fluid nature of, 1–2
  as generalizations, 124
  as guidelines, 2, 17
  Hippocratic Oath, founded on, 4
  justice, 88–90
  lifestyle choices, 180–181
  non-maleficence *see* non-maleficence
  respect, 83
ethics
  duty-based, and deontology, 189–190
  ethical theories and natural justice,
    192–194
  and legal obligations, 192
  meaning, 1–3
  morality, conflict with, 181–183
    see also morality
  normative, in health care, 194
  practice of, 188–189
  practice rules/regulations, 186
  proactive nature of, 88
  and society, 197–198
  virtue, 194–195
ethics-paternalism, and society, 197–198
euthanasia, 71, 72, 198–199
examinations
  inadequate, 40
  intraocular pressure, glaucoma,
    57–58, 69
  time for, 51
exemplary behaviour, optometrists,
    35, 37

F

F v West Berkshire Health Authority,
    mentally incompetent adult case,
    76–77
factual causation, breach of duty of
    care, 148–151
fair trial, right to, 124
fairness, 14
Family Law Reform Act 1969, 65
fixed-term contracts, discrimination, 137
floaters, case study, 93
football players, contrasted with
    doctors, 20
forgiveness, 16
forseeability test, remoteness, 151

free will, and morality, 189
freedom of choice *see* autonomy
freedom of thought, ethical requirement, 202–203
functionalist approach to profession definition, 30

G

General Medical Council, guidance on information to patients, 68
General Ophthalmic Services (GOS), 172
General Optical Council (GOC), 35
generalizations, 124–125
Gillick v West Norfolk and Wisbech Area Health Authority, 74–76
   Gillick competency, and children under 16 years, 75, 119
glasses *see* spectacles
glaucoma
   failure to diagnose, 153
   family history of, 57
   risks, informing patients about, 69
   up to date knowledge requirement, 39
GOC (General Optical Council), 35
good deeds, and ethical behaviour, 1, 49–50
   see also beneficence
GOS (General Ophthalmic Services), 172
'greater good', distributing resources according to, 99–100
Green, Phillip, 193
grievances claims, 38
gross professional misconduct, 40–41

H

happiness, and utilitarianism, 190
harassment
   age discrimination, 137
   Protection from Harassment Act 1997, 138
   racial discrimination, 134
   sex discrimination, 133
   sexual orientation discrimination, 137
harm
   see also non-maleficence
   avoidance, 15
   breach of duty of care, resulting from, 148–151
   prevention of

harm *(Continued)*
      as act of beneficence or non-maleficence, 62–63
      role of patient, 59–62
   self-harm or harm to others, protecting patient from, 107–109
   case studies, 53–54, 56, 107-109
Haw, Brian, 202
Health and Safety at Work etc Act 1974, 138
health and safety factors, optometric code, 35
hedonism, 9, 167
Heinz' dilemma, Kohlberg's moral reasoning stages, 12, 13
Hippocrates, 4, 6, 19, 60, 62
Hippocratic Oath
   beneficence principle, 49
   confidentiality requirements, 38, 103
   cosmetic surgery, 182
   and Declaration of Geneva (Physician's Oath) 1948, 7
   ethical principles founded on, 4
   history of ethics, 5–6
   and modern ethical codes, 6
   non-maleficence principle, 57
   professionalization of medicine, 19
   version of, 5–6
Human Rights Act 1998, 71, 72, 81, 82

I

idealistic motives, profession choice, 24, 25
illegality, and morality, 16
individual rights, balancing against societal good, 88
Information Commissioner, 115, 116
information disclosure *see* disclosures
information transfer, healthcare disclosures, 118
injuries, caused by negligence, 149, 152
institutions, and ethics, 6
insurance, professional, 35–36
integrity, 16, 39–40
intraocular pressure, glaucoma examination, 57–58, 69
in-vitro fertilization (IVF) treatment, ethical decisions, 54, 55–56

J

Jehovah's Witnesses, 76
Johnson, Samuel, 19
journalism, and profession, 23
judgement, 90–95
    information needed to make, 91–93
    trust in, 93–95
justice, 85–102
    and beneficence, 181
    case studies, 91–92, 93
    corrective, 95
    distributive see resource distribution
    as ethical principle, 88–90
    fair trial, right to, 124
    judgement, 90–95, 91–93
    legal see legal justice
    natural, and ethical theories, 192–194
    Robin Hood approach to, 184

K

Kant, Immanuel, 1, 189, 192
keratoconus, 61
King, Gregory, 19
Kohlberg, Lawrence
    moral reasoning stages of, 12, 13
Kouao, Marie-Thérèse, 111, 112, 113

L

laser surgery, refractive errors, 168, 182
law
    confidentiality in, 113–121
    and deontology, 192
    ethics, conflict with, 183–186
    fair trial, right to, 124
    justice see justice; legal justice
    and morals, 16
    vs. natural justice, 192–193
    of obligations, 142
learned professional, 29–30
legal justice, 85–88
    see also justice; law
    adjustments, need for, 87
    application of, variation in, 86
    crime and punishment, 86
    Disability Discrimination Act 1995, 87
    individual rights, balancing against societal good, 88
    limitations, 88
liberty rights, 44

life and death decisions, 175–176
lifestyle choices, ethical principles, 180–181
Limitation Act 1980, 157–158
love, protection based on, 200–202

M

macular degeneration, 14
Majrowski, William, 138–139
malignant disease, 73, 153, 178
management, and profession, 23
management ethics and social responsibility, 165–166
manipulation, in advertising, 168
Manning, Carl, 111
manual data, 116
married couples, respecting confidentiality of, 119–120
materialistic motives, profession choice, 24, 25
medical intervention, lifestyle choices, 50–51
Medicines and Healthcare Products Regulatory Agency (MHRA), 118
merit or achievement, resource distribution, 97–98
meta-ethics, 188
Metaphysics of Ethics (Kant), 189
MHRA (Medicines and Healthcare Products Regulatory Agency), 118
Mill, John Stuart, 65, 190, 197
misconduct, 40–41, 126
MMR vaccine, encouragement for, 198
morality, 9–15
    and autonomy, 189
    case study, 10–11
    doing one's best, 15
    ethics, conflict with, 181–183
    fairness, 14
    fluid nature of, 11–12
    and free will, 189
    harm, avoidance, 15
    health care, moral code in, 14
    Heinz' dilemma, 12–13
    Kohlberg's moral reasoning stages, 12, 13
    law and morals, 16
    multifactorial factors influencing, 11
    patient's decisions, respecting, 15
    religious beliefs, 10–11, 12

Mother Teresa, as beneficient person, 52
myopia, correction, 58–59, 180

N

National Health Service (NHS)
　contracts with, 171–172
　limited resources of, 97
　Litigation Authority Journal, 158
need, resource distribution, 96–97
negligence, 142–159
　case studies
　　Bolam v Friern Hospital Manage-
　　　ment Committee, 145–146, 147
　　Bolitho v City and Hackney
　　　Health Authority, 147
　　Donoghue v Stevenson,
　　　142, 143–144
　　Fairchild v Glenhaven Funeral
　　　Services Ltd and Others, 149
　　Smith v Tunbridge Wells Health
　　　Authority, 148
　conditions to prove, 143
　damages claims, practitioner
　　protection, 154
　duty of care see duty of care
　failure to diagnose a serious disease
　　or condition, 153
　failure to inform about a condition,
　　152–153
　injuries caused by, 149, 152
　potential for in primary eye care
　　practice, 152–153
　record keeping, importance, 154–158
　vicarious liability, 158–159
neighbour principle, tort law, 144
NHS see National Health Service
　(NHS)
Niyazov, Saparmurat (President of
　Turkmenistan), 9, 10
non-maleficence
　and autonomy, 70
　and beneficence, 57
　　see also beneficence
　harm, prevention of, 59–62, 62–63
　integral to clinical practice, 63
　judging of, 179
　limits, 64
　patient, role of, 59–62
　risks and benefits, analysis, 57–59

normative ethical practice, 188
normative ethics, in health care, 194
Northern Ireland, racial discrimination
　legislation, 133

O

obesity
　childhood, 82
　disease risk, 96
　in-vitro fertilization (IVF) treatment,
　　refusal of, 56
　medical intervention, 50
　state intervention, 199
obligations, law of, 142
offer and acceptance, contract law, 169,
　170–171
ophthalmoscopy, cancer detection, 178
optometric code of ethics, 33–42
　see also optometrists
　American Optometric Association, 34
　ethical concepts see ethical concepts
　guiding principles, 35–42
　health and safety factors, 35
　as series of guidelines, 41
optometrists
　see also optometric code of ethics
　behaviour standards expected, 35
　commercial side of practice, 163
　competition between practices, 125
　co-operation, need for, 40
　examinations, inadequate, 40
　gross professional misconduct, 40–41
　junior and senior, relationships
　　between, 123
　larger practices, 38–39, 163
　law, up to date knowledge
　　requirement, 38
　limitations of some, 41
　practice management, 38, 39–40
　practitioner-patient relationship,
　　trust issues, 94
　relationships between see collegiality
　small or single practitioner practices,
　　38, 163
　specialist status, retention of, 41
optometry
　code of ethics see optometric code of
　　ethics
　motives, profession choice, 25–26

optometry (*Continued*)
  as profession, 33
  success, measuring, 28
Oracles, 19
orthokeratology
  limitations of some optometrists, 41
  myopia, correction, 58–59
  risks, 180

P

PARN (Professional Associations Research profession), 23
part-time workers, discrimination against, 137
paternalism
  defined, 197
  in health care, 198–199
  9/11 terrorist attacks, 198
  society and ethics, 197–198
patient choices
  business ethics, 163–165
  consumer choices compared, 164
  respect for, 15, 69–71
patients
  see also patient choices
  and customers, 162–163
  desires of, acting or not acting in accordance with, 54, 55–56, 168
  duties of doctors to, 8, 122
  elderly, communication with, 77–78
  failure to diagnose a serious disease or condition, 153
  failure to inform about a condition, 152–153
  informing about condition and treatment, 59–62
  informing about risks, 68–69
  new, and trust issues, 94
  non-English speaking, 134–135
  recollections of procedures, 156
  role of, in prevention of harm, 59–62
  vulnerable *see* vulnerable patients
Percival, Thomas, 6
personal data, 113, 118
  handling, 114–115
personality differences, in health care, 196–197
philosophy and ethical theory, 188–203
  deontology, 189–190, 191, 192, 194

philosophy and ethical theory (*Continued*)
  means or ends, 189–191
  natural justice, 192–194
  normative ethics, in health care, 194
  practice of ethics, 188–189
  society and ethics, 197–198
  utilitarianism, 190–191, 192, 194
  virtue ethics, 194–195
    in health care, 195–197
Physician's Oath (Declaration of Geneva) 1948, 7
Piaget, Jean, 12
politicians, and profession, 23
positive discrimination, 137
power, and approach to profession definitions, 30
practice management, 38, 39–40
practice rules/regulations, and ethics, 186
practitioner-patient relationship
  ethical principles, 122
  husband and wife, 120
  trust issues, 94
prejudice, and collegiality, 125
premises, insurance of, 36
Pretty, Diane, 72
problem recognition, collegiality, 126–129
productivity, resource distribution, 98–99
professio, meaning, 30
profession
  see also professions
  choice of, motives, 24–26
  definitions, 29, 30, 31
    modern meaning, 20–24
  discrediting of members, 40
  obligation to practise ethically, 24
  optometry as, 33
Professional Associations Research Network (PARN), 23
professional compromise, 117
professions
  see also profession
  behaviour expected from professionals, 35, 36, 37
  future of, 29–30
  history and development, 19–20

professions (*Continued*)
  other occupations distinguished,
    21–24
  success, measuring, 26–29
  trades distinguished, 21
profit-making, and business ethics,
  162, 163, 165
prolonging of treatment, and
  compassion, 53
public interest, resource distribution,
  99–100

R

racial discrimination
  in healthcare practice, 134–135
  religion or faith, 135
  statutory provisions, 133, 134, 135
Rashbrook, Patricia, 54, 55–56
realistic motives, profession choice,
  24, 25
reason, and ethical behaviour, 1
record keeping, importance, 154–158
  guidelines, 155–156
  retention of records, 157–158
recruitment practices, and judgement, 91
referrals, sharing of patient
  information, 118
Reformation, 162
refractive surgery, 58–59, 180
refusal of treatment, 56, 73–74, 177
religious beliefs 10–11, 12
  lack of, 90
religious discrimination, 135
remoteness, breach of duty of care, 151
resource distribution, 95–102
  according to effort and sacrifice,
    97–98
  according to merit or achievement,
    97–98
  according to need, 96–97
  according to productivity, 98–99
  according to public interest or
    greater good, 99–100
  according to usefulness in society or
    supply scarcity, 100–102
  canons of, 95, 101
  case study, 101
  equal, 96
  and lifestyle choices, 180

respect, ethical concepts, 44–45
Respect for Private and Family Life,
  81
responsibility, 16, 46
retinal detachment, 153, 158–159
rights, ethical concepts, 44
risks, patient information, 68–69
Road Traffic Act 1988, 117
Ross, William David, 52
Royal College of Physicians, 30, 31
Royal Society for the Promotion of
  Health, 23
Ruhnama (Book of the Soul), 9

S

salaries and wages, variation in,
  97–98
schizophrenia, 77
sensitive personal data, 113, 118
  prescription as, 120
sex discrimination, 132–133
sexism, in workplace, 127–129
sexual harassment, 133
sexual orientation, discrimination,
  136–137
short-sightedness *see* myopia, correction
Sidaway v Board of Governors, 68
sight-threatening decisions, 3–4
single practitioner practices,
  confidentiality requirements, 38
smoking
  as dangerous lifestyle habit, 82, 180
  and diabetic retinopathy, 51, 70
  medical intervention, 50–51
snakes, healing rituals, 4
Snellen chart, 58
social responsibility, and management
  ethics, 165–166
Socrates, 9
spectacles
  advertising of, 168
  driving, needed for, 194
  incorrect prescription, injury caused
    by, 149
myopia, correction, 58–59, 180
  prescription changes, 2, 15
standards, ethical concepts, 46
state intervention, paternalism,
  198–199

success, measuring, 26–29
supply scarcity, resource distribution, 100–102

T

tax, obligation to pay, 193
teaching and medicine, recognition of, 27
teleology, 190–191, 194
temp test, manual data, 116
terminal illness, 72, 198–199
Opticians Act 1989 (Amendment) Order 2005, 35
tonometry, 69, 152
tort, 142–143
trade, profession distinguished, 21
traditional ethical practice, 188
traits of character, professionals, 30, 196
trust, 93–95, 104
tumours, 73, 153, 178

U

unbearable suffering, defined, 72
United Nations Universal Declaration of Human Rights, 101
unmarried fathers, and right to know, 120–121
usefulness, resource distribution,, 100–102
utilitarianism
  deontology contrasted, 191
  and teleology, 190–191
  virtue ethics, 194

V

values, ethical concepts, 43–44
vegetative states, and life support decisions, 177

vexatious litigant, damages claims, 154
vicarious liability, 150, 158–159
victimization
  age discrimination, 137
  bullying at work, 139
  gender-based discrimination, 132–133
  racial discrimination, 134
  sexual orientation discrimination, 137
virtue ethics, 194–195
  in health care, 195–197
virtues, ethical concepts, 43
vitreous detachment, 93
vulnerable patients
  see also children
  College of Optometrists on, 106
  description, 106
  elderly patients, 78
  protection, 200–202
    and confidentiality, 106–107
  rights of, 81–83

W

War Crimes, 7
'whole world', offers to, 169–170
World Medical Association (WMA), International Code of Medical Ethics, 7–8
Wyatt, Charlotte, 4–5, 97

Z

Zeus, 4